MW01174847

December 1999.

HEARTS AND FLOWERS

June Buckley

MINERVA PRESS
MONTREUX   LONDON   WASHINGTON

HEARTS AND FLOWERS
Copyright © June Buckley 1996

All Rights Reserved

ISBN 1 86106 006 8

First Published 1996 by
MINERVA PRESS
195 Knightsbridge,
London SW7 1RE

Printed in Great Britain by
B.W.D. Ltd, Northolt, Middlesex.

HEARTS AND FLOWERS

To my husband and family, and the medics who helped me.

Before

"That's it then. Finish. Out."

These words greeted me on a visit to the doctor's surgery on April 16th 1986, before morning school. I just stared at the doctor, unable to believe him, and muttered, "But I can't."

"Why? Is it the money?"

"No, not really, but I can't switch off mentally, just like that," I replied.

"In that case, go back to school and before you do anything else see George [the headmaster] and tell him that you've to do nothing else except teach."

Slowly I walked to the school wondering how ill I really was. How much longer would I be able to walk across the recreation ground? How much longer would I live?

I knocked on the headmaster's door and at his, "Come in," I walked in and immediately burst into tears. Very calmly the head told me to sit down while he made quite a fuss washing his hands in the adjoining cloakroom. He then left the room, returning a few minutes later with a tray of coffee.

"Now, can you tell me what's wrong?" he asked.

I explained what the doctor had told me, stating that I did not want a lot of fuss made or my poor health to become public knowledge. George just sat and listened. Looking back, I think the doctor, who was also a school governor, had probably forewarned the head.

The deputy head had to be informed because of the various duty lists which would have to be rearranged. No more detention or bus duties for me! However, when it came to giving up my position as Head of House, I refused, saying that I enjoyed it and would carry on. I didn't regard the weekly assembly for some two hundred and fifty, or more pupils and staff to be stressful, having taken assemblies for a number of years. That meant that I still continued in my weekly general duty to support the house prefects. Various house matches also needed supporting. I continued with parents' evenings, as how could I teach and not see parents?

I had stopped attending out-of-school meetings after a young man had told me, in front of many teaching colleagues, that I could not possibly be going into ordinary classes to help special needs pupils who for one reason or another could not cope, as the idea had only just been thought up.

"But I've been doing that for years," I protested. He said he did not believe me. After being called a liar, I decided that enough was enough regarding so-called experts and their meetings. The old adage 'there's nothing new under the sun,' comes to mind!

That fateful April doctor's visit came after I had undergone various X-rays and ECGs at the local hospital.

I suppose it all began when my ankles started swelling, which made me realise that something was amiss. For some time I had become breathless running upstairs, bouncing on the trampoline or climbing hills. Living in the centre of the Pennines, hills were a real problem. I had dismissed all this as 'growing older'. However, the ankle oedema was something else, so I finally sought medical help at the end of February 1986. After a course of diuretics, shape returned to my ankles, but as soon as the effect of the drugs wore off the oedema returned, hence the need for the tests, and the shattering news from the doctor.

A visit to the consultant cardiologist had spelt out the exact diagnosis. I had an enlarged heart, an irregular heartbeat, congested lungs, excess fluid and cardiomyapathy. I was told to go home and rest for a month. Rest! Me? When I asked if could have a pub lunch, the consultant said, "I said *home and rest!*" The pub lunch won. It was much easier having that than going home to cook!

Thus started regular hospital visits for tests and drugs. I returned to teaching, even though Alan, my husband, had been given early retirement. For many years we had taught at the same comprehensive school, through which our three children had passed. I had always thought that I was known there as Alan's wife, or Cheryl, Alison or Chris's mother and I wanted to be 'me' instead. Therefore I continued working for a further two years, having numerous chest clinic appointments and absences from school.

At every hospital visit, the cardiologist asked the same two questions, "How many pillows do you use? Do you do your own housework?"

I always replied, "None," and, "Not if I can help it."

Finally, in answer to the second question I answered, "I work full-time, my husband is retired and I have a superb cleaning lady, so I would be a fool to do my own housework." The consultant never asked me those questions again.

During this time I had agreed to start a trial drug procedure, which meant even more hospital visits and working on the exercise bicycle. In spite of saying that I came from Norfolk, where cycling was easier because of the lack of hills, the pedals were regularly tightened to make pedalling harder. I never managed more than nine and a half minutes on the exercise bicycle and I never found out anything about the trial drug either.

I sent in my resignation in March 1988, two years after I had been told to finish teaching. The end of my career came in July. I can well remember the headmaster telling me that when the Chief Education Officer came to the school I was expected to go to the school office so that he could say goodbye to me.

I refused, saying, "If the Chief Education Officer could not see me when I was teaching, I certainly don't want to see him when I am leaving."

The fact that on the day of the visit I was once again at the chest clinic made my controversial decision much simpler.

So began my retirement. Much of the early time was spent in the garden, both working and relaxing. I decided to do some voluntary work at the local Physically Handicapped and Able Bodied Club as they were appealing for help. To begin with, there were three of us who had volunteered, all strangers to each other. After the third weekly visit, one lady said, "I don't think I can come anymore. I only have one lung."

Joan, never short of anything to say, was the next to say, "I'm all right, but I only have one kidney."

It was my turn then. "I've a weak heart." There we were, helping the disabled!

Acting on the suggestions made by various House staff members that I should have my assemblies published, I started sorting out, collating and writing out eleven years of those assemblies which I deemed suitable for further reading. This occupied much of my spare time during the autumn and winter days of my newfound leisure time. When my daughter and son-in-law asked who I would ask to publish the work with, I said, "I don't know, probably someone like Longman's, the educational publishers."

At this they both said, "No, it should be a general publisher so that a greater audience would be reached." Alison continued with, "I always listen to the car radio as I'm driving to work, and your assembly themes would suit something like the 'Thought For Today' programme."

Tony volunteered to send my work to such a publisher which he duly did. However, I've heard nothing further, so I assume that the script was either lost or thought unsuitable. Maybe I'll try again sometime.

Reassembling the 'talks' kept me occupied for a considerable time, which was all to the good. I had a few ex-pupils who needed some extra English tuition, or rather whose parents had requested it, so they came along for hourly sessions after school. I enjoyed this and hope they did not regard it as too much of an imposition.

It was suggested that I put in a claim for a disability pension, so I applied for this at the beginning of 1989.

A visit to the Medical Board of Assessment was necessary. This was an extremely humiliating experience. I walked into a meeting room and sat facing two doctors, on one side of a large paper-strewn table.

The condescending voice of the woman doctor was unpleasant to say the least, as she asked various questions, probing my ability to do household tasks. Her tone altered somewhat when I handed over a written list detailing things I could no longer do, such as rubbing myself dry and carrying anything slightly weighty. When I was examined by the male doctor, he commented to his compatriot on my heartbeat with, "Come and listen to this, I've never heard anything like it. It's like an express train going over the points."

This would have terrified someone of a nervous disposition! I was feeling very unwell at the time, otherwise I would have complained about their attitude and general behaviour. Two days after this examination, I was in the local hospital having over a litre of fluid removed from a lung.

This was a frightening experience, as three nurses came into the room followed by the consultant and a doctor. I sat straddled over a chair, and two nurses held my arms which were folded across the back of the chair. The consultant showed his companion where to probe my back and then left the room.

The procedure was not explained to me at all. I was merely told to sit still, which I did until the last of the fluid was sucked out of my lung, and I shot out of the chair. The noise made was similar to the noise from the last drop of liquid being drawn up through a straw.

A few days after this I was back home again, having spent the first of several stays in hospital. As a first experience, except for hospital stays for births, it was quite pleasant. As the ward was being decorated, the private wing was taken over and I had a single room, which was nicely furnished and carpeted. The food was attractively presented and well cooked. The nursing staff were friendly and cheerful and I was free to wander around serving teas, collecting cups, and talking to patients.

Some days after my return home I received the results of the Medical Board's examination, which stated that I was sixty percent disabled. I could not claim for disability allowance as the criterion was eighty percent. However, I could appeal, which I did. While waiting to hear the date of the medical tribunal, I continued living as normally as possible.

The second Saturday in June was the local old people's tea and entertainment in the village, and as usual I spent the day working there, preparing and serving the food.

The following lunchtime, Alan and I decided to have a pub lunch at a local hostelry just over the Lancashire border. After one mouthful of delicious roast ham, I blacked out. The next thing I remember is an ambulanceman bending over me. I managed to get into a wheelchair, and then the frightening ambulance journey began. Alan followed by car and later told me that we were travelling at over seventy miles an hour, with horn blaring and lights flashing. I braced myself with my feet on the seat opposite and clung to the arms of the chair.

I asked the cheery ambulanceman how many patients they lost on their way to hospital!

My treatment in the Rochdale hospital was quick, thorough and friendly. Soon Alan and I were on our way home – lunchless! What a thing to do in a crowded pub.

We have been back to that public house a few times since my transplant and enjoyed their excellent value meals. They remembered me!

The medical tribunal was another unpleasant occasion. This time the walk from the door to the much larger table was further than before and there were three interrogators. The result, received a month later, was the same as before – sixty percent disabled. This time the letter stated that there was no further appeal allowed, unless there was a legal loophole.

Thanks to my GP, I could appeal to the commissioner's office in London, as there *was* a legal loophole. I had not been examined by a cardiac specialist: the examiners were general and orthopaedic surgeons.

I delayed writing to the commissioner's office, mainly because I was back in hospital – the newly-decorated ward this time, but the same nursing staff. There was an extra probationer nurse, who had been a pupil at school until the previous July. Staff generally called patients by their first name. That young nurse studiously declined to call me anything.

One of the patients was a large, cheerful lady, who had been advised to lose weight. Anyone who has been in hospital and had an operation, however minor, will know that the garment given to the patient to wear is a cotton shift, which is open all the way down the back. If the recipient is lucky, there will be enough tapes at the neck, halfway down the back, and waist, to enable the garment to be tied, providing some decorum.

This patient, the cheerful, large lady, was given a garment which barely covered her knees and was not wide enough to enable her to tie the tapes. Fortunately she saw the funny side.

A few hours later, when it was my turn to don a 'designer' gown, it trailed on the floor and wrapped round me twice.

One evening the lady asked her husband at visiting time if he would bring in some more knickers for her. She told him exactly where they were, stressing which drawer and which side of the drawer in her dressing table these garments were kept. She was not at all amused the following evening when her husband duly arrived with three pairs of his underpants. He argued that they would fit her and said that he had not been able to find any knickers. We were all highly amused.

My drugs were altered once again and I underwent the usual tests. I was even allowed home for a few hours on Sunday. This was good, as weekends in hospital are somewhat deadly – nothing happens.

I did experience one new examination. The people of Halifax and district had donated enough money to buy a CT scanner. The examination on that narrow, hard table and the movement backwards and forwards, in and out of the 'upturned hairdryer hood' took over three-quarters of an hour. The radiologists' instructions every few seconds to "Hold your breath", followed by "Breathe normally" almost sent me into a hypnotic trance.

Before this stay in hospital we had planned a visit to our daughter in Oxfordshire and I had booked a day at Fartheringhoe for Alison and me to attend a cookery demonstration. I begged the consultant to discharge me, and one patient said that she had never heard anyone plead so eloquently.

One of my arguments was that my son-in-law was a doctor, so I would be in good hands. It worked, and by late morning we were on our way.

All went well until south of Leicester, when we encountered fog which became denser the further we travelled. We found that Alison was not at home. She had taken Macsen, her son, to the doctor and was delayed by the fog too. Tony, her husband, should have been flying back from Italy: the fog was to blame again. The Italian airport would not answer Alison's numerous phone calls on her return home and London said that always happened in a crisis, such as fog. Alison had no idea where Tony was and she was becoming more and more worried, particularly as there had been no phone call from Tony either. As we were waiting anxiously, there was an almighty crash. Hannis, the large English pointer dog, had fallen down the stairs in the throes of an epileptic fit. All he wanted was for Alison to stroke his head and hold his paw. So much for me being in good hands!

By the next morning, the fog had cleared, Tony had arrived, and the cookery demonstration was very enjoyable.

In December I wrote to the commissioner's office about the disability claim, and there was a long delay before an answer was received, or rather an acknowledgement of my letter.

The beginning of 1990 saw a further deterioration in my health. The effects of one of the drugs gave me diarrhoea and a rash which was extremely itchy. I scratched my back and shoulders in my sleep and regularly had a blood-speckled nightdress. I delayed going to the doctor, but eventually I had to succumb, the result was that I was once again back in the infirmary. I began to feel like a regular visitor; one of the nurses said that it was time a bed was reserved for me.

In the six-bedded bay we had a jolly time. It is surprising how sometimes everyone gels and gets on together, and this was one such occasion. We were regularly reprimanded for laughing too much. We talked and talked and still keep in touch. Being in someone's company for twenty-fours a day, every day, is not normal. I chatted to one of the male nurses in particular for considerable periods of time, but more about him later.

On February 16th 1990, the consultant dropped his bombshell. It was his usual bi-weekly ward visit with his entourage. After a brief examination of my bedside notes and me, he said that I could go home that evening. Then in a loud voice he said, "Lie back, I want to ask you something – what do you think about a heart transplant?"

The attendant staff nurse gasped and I stared at him before blurting out, "B-but I'm not ill enough."

I had only heard of heart transplants being done when a patient only had a few days to live, and when there were appeals on the media for donors.

The consultant then said, "I would like you to go home this evening and talk it over with your family, then come back here in three days' time with your decision."

As I've mentioned, the consultant had spoken quite loudly, and within minutes everyone on the ward knew the news. I spoke to the staff nurse who had gasped, and she said how surprised she was, as I was the last person in the ward she would have expected to be given that news.

Alan came to visit me as usual that evening and I was ready to go home. While I was at the nurses' station collecting my tablets, one of the patients told Alan about the transplant news. That should never have happened.

On the way home I chattered about everything except the transplant. As soon as we were indoors, and after one of his numerous cups of coffee, Alan went upstairs for a bath. I phoned the doctor at home and asked if he could come and see me the next day; I did not want to go to the surgery.

"Can you tell me what it is about?" he asked.

"Don't you know?"

"You tell me," he said. I did. His reply was that it had been on the cards for some time. He would come and see me after his morning surgery.

When Alan came downstairs, I told him that the doctor was coming the next morning and that a heart transplant had been suggested. Alan's comment was that he already knew and that he had been expecting that news long before he had been told so uncaringly that evening in the hospital.

I said that I would telephone our three children, but that the decision had to be mine. If a transplant was offered, I would jump at the chance. I phoned and told the children my decision. A few days before this, Alison had booked a holiday in a gîte in Brittany for her two children, our two Canadian grandsons, and us. We had been looking forward to hearing how Montreal French coped with French. That holiday was cancelled, which meant the loss of the deposit.

The doctor came after his surgery and stayed for nearly an hour answering my questions.

I asked if I could be put in touch with someone who had undergone a heart transplant, but he said, "Sorry, I don't know anyone!"

After three days I returned to the hospital and said that I was prepared to have a transplant if it was feasible. The consultant said that he would send my notes and a covering letter to Leeds General Infirmary that day, and I would be transferred to that hospital.

It wasn't until many months later that I learnt it was my GP who had persuaded the consultant to consider me for transplantation. The consultant had said that I was too old, to which Malcolm (my GP) had replied, "Rubbish! You don't know her." How glad I am that Malcolm knew me!

At about this time, the long-awaited and extremely long-winded reply came from the commissioner's office stating that I could appeal against the tribunal's findings. The language used was difficult to understand and the sentences were so long and complicated that we decided to ask a solicitor for his advice and help. At the same time we also made our wills.

The first visit to the General Infirmary in Leeds came in early April when I attended the surgeon's clinic. Despite being such a large bustling hospital, it had a friendly atmosphere and the surgeon was so courteous and down-to-earth that the whole occasion was worry-free. Arrangements were made for me to become an in-patient at the hospital so that an assessment could be made as to my suitability for transplantation.

I was still going to the Calder Valley Disabled Club on a weekly basis and told the manager my news, but I asked her to keep it quiet. However, she did tell the chairman, which was to be expected. Very quietly this lady came up to me and asked if I knew anyone who had had a transplant, and would I like to talk to someone. I said that I had asked the doctor to put me in touch with a transplantee but that he knew no one.

I was given a telephone number, and a few days later Alan and I drove over the moors to Keighley to meet Jo and her husband Phil.

Jo is very special to us. Just after I had first met her I mentioned that the consultant I saw in Leeds was Dr Smith. Jo asked me to describe him, which I did. She then exclaimed, "He's *my* Dr Smith," and went on to explain that as a child she had had a congenital heart problem, and when she had been in her early teens, her mother had asked for a second opinion concerning Jo's condition. They were sent to London where Jo was seen by a Dr Smith, who told her that the only thing which would help her was a heart and lung transplant. As that was over twenty years ago, it had been unavailable. Nine years ago, Jo had the operation and now helps counsel others both before and after their transplants. Jo is almost the longest surviving heart-and-lung transplantee in the world. What a wonderful achievement!

We soon became friends with Jo and her husband and still meet regularly. From being confined to a wheelchair Jo now tackles hills in the Lake District, goes skiing, and participates in the Transplant Games which are held annually.

She contacted Dr Smith and he was delighted to hear that his prognosis had come true.

Assessment time arrived and I was told that I would be in hospital for approximately five days, undergoing a battery of tests. On arriving at the cardiothoracic ward, I was allocated a bed in the small, four-bedded side ward, with two male and two female patients. This was my first experience of a mixed ward.

Tests started the next day when a number of blood samples were taken, and also the following tests: X-ray, ECG, echo cardiograph, lung function, ultrasound, saliva, urine, angiography, and biopsy. All these took several days, and the five days stretched to twelve days. The main reason for the length of stay was because the first biopsy was not successful. I had become very uncomfortable during the angiography so the biopsy needed to be redone. The hospital had exhausted their supply of special catheters, so I had to wait until more could be obtained.

The sound of blood passing round the heart during the echo cardiograph was amazing, and I commented that if my washing machine sounded like that I would be panicking. During the ultrasound tests the technician remarked that I had a beautiful spleen. I lay there thinking, "Blow my spleen, it's my kidneys and liver I'm concerned about!"

A hospital social worker came and talked about my interests, the type of house I lived in, who would be able to look after me, and so on. She also asked me how I felt about having someone else's heart. I replied that for years I carried a donor card, so if I was prepared to give I should also be prepared to receive. The ward sister also questioned me about having someone else's organ.

Apart from all the physical tests there were five criteria to fulfil also: to be thinnish, a non-smoker, non-alcoholic, fit, apart from the heart, and positive. Thankfully, all of these I passed.

In many ways I welcomed the longer stay on the cardiothorocic ward because I met Ken. Ken had undergone a successful heart transplant two days before I went into hospital. When he was able to have visitors in his single room, I spent several hours sitting on his bed and talking to him. Ken did my confidence a power of good.

The weather during this time was extremely hot, so patients and their visitors spent a great deal of time wandering in the garden which was quite delightful. Ken used to join us too, as did all the smokers. At night our room was like a greenhouse and sleeping in bed became a problem.

The occupants of the room altered, sometimes daily. It was used mainly for those awaiting a bypass operation or valve replacement and for those almost ready for home after an operation. I was the odd one out.

Some people are remembered more than others. Sam was a delightful man, very cheerful and always smiling. I said to him one day, "Your watch has a very loud tick." He laughed, and pointing to his watch, said, "It doesn't work. The ticking is my new heart valve!"

There was the country and western singer who used to entertain in local Leeds pubs. He was terrified of his impending bypass operation. My female companion at that time was an excellent singer, so we passed several hours singing various songs. I say 'we' but most of the singing was done by the other two while I did embroidery or knitting. The man – I have forgotten his name now – had a demonstration tape of his singing brought in for Janette to listen to. Janette suggested that he had it reproduced with a better guitar accompaniment, as the singing was good but not the strumming. I said that if that was done we could say that we knew him before he became well known. Back came the retort, "You can also say that you slept with me."

We had an evening's amusement at Malcolm's expense. He came in for a heart bypass operation, and prior to the morning's surgery it was necessary to shave his legs and chest. Veins from the legs are generally used to bypass the damaged or clotted arteries of the heart. Two razors were brought to Malcolm and he retired behind his bed curtains.

At frequent intervals Malcolm's head would peep through the curtains and ask someone for more razors. This scenario continued for over two hours, until either eleven or thirteen razors had been supplied. We were curious to know what was happening, when finally Malcolm drew back the curtains and with a huge sigh of relief announced, "I've *finished.*"

The sister, with an absolutely straight face, looked at him and said, "What about your moustache?" The look of horror on his face had us almost in hysterics before Malcolm realised that she was joking.

Unfortunately, his operation did not take place the next day as there was an emergency and then the surgeon was away for two weeks. Malcolm was sent home for a fortnight. I often wonder if he repeated the shaving pantomime all over again! I do know, though, that the bypass operation was successful when it eventually happened.

One sad event occurred at this time. Annie, a tortoise which we had had for twenty-eight years, died. She was quite a character and had been brought for Cheryl, our elder daughter, when she was seven years old. She had been christened Annigoni by Cheryl because she liked the sound of the name. Annie had led an eventful life, one way and another

She had been trodden on once, on her head, and for some time after that she was disorientated and would walk around in small circles. She had once been stolen from the pen in the garden, and in spite of making exhaustive enquiries around the locality no one knew anything about Annie's whereabouts.

By pure accident, a couple of weeks after her disappearance, I had taken my class to Heptonstall, the old historic village nearby, and rather than return to school after our visit, the pupils were allowed home. One boy said that he was going to his sister's house as she had found a tortoise and did not want it.

Keith was going to have it. I was curious and asked him to bring the tortoise to me. When he did, I was delighted to recognise Annie – her head had an indentation from being trodden on, so she was easily recognised.

There was no way that Annie could have climbed down the garden steps and wandered over a mile uphill to where she was 'found'.

On another occasion, I used Annie as an illustration in a House assembly. The theme of the assembly was: 'Things aren't what they always appear to be'. I commented on the name Annigoni, saying that to most people, Annigoni was a famous Italian artist but to our family it meant our tortoise. Bending down, I picked Annie out of my basket to show the pupils and she immediately urinated on the floor.

Quelling the smirking pupils in front of me, I soon dissolved into fits of giggling myself when one small boy whispered loudly, "I'm glad it wasn't an elephant, miss!" When I meet these pupils now, although they are quite grown up, they always remember the tortoise assembly.

I was very sad when Alan brought me the news of Annie's death.

A few evenings prior to the second biopsy, the consultant and registrar came to my bed, greatly excited. The Pathology Department thought that mast cells had been found in my heart. When I asked what that meant, I was told that if it were so, a heart transplant would *not* be carried out, as mast cells would infiltrate a new heart.

They then said that enquiries would have to be made somewhere in America where research had been carried out on this rare happening. How relieved I was to discover that mast cells were *not* present after further tests on my heart. After the second biopsy I returned home.

Towards the end of May, I was asked back to the cardiologist's clinic where the registrar told me that a heart transplant was strongly recommended, and if I was agreeable a further appointment would be made for me to see the surgeon. Three days later we were back at the hospital where the surgeon said that I would be put on the transplant waiting lists from that day – 22nd May 1990.

The pros and cons were spelt out by the friendly, gentlemanly young surgeon and I was told that no one else with my blood group was waiting. As I belong to the common 'A positive' group I felt hopeful about an early call. When I asked how long I would have to wait, the surgeon shrugged his shoulders and said, "Two days, two weeks, two months."

Happily, I returned home to wait.

The Waiting

The next morning I contacted British Telecom to enquire about a radio pager which would enable me to go beyond hearing distance of the telephone. Some hospitals supply these 'bleepers' for transplant patients but not Leeds. However, BT waived the connecting charge and said that as soon as they had received my cheque for three months rental a pager would be dispatched.

The pager duly arrived and I felt free to go to the village and to places within the pager's radius from the hospital, which was twenty-five miles. We lived twenty-two and a half miles away, so excursions west were limited, but otherwise I was not really aware of being restricted too much.

I am positive that the pager was designed by a man with men's clothing in mind. The pager would clip conveniently on to a trouser belt or pocket and could easily be carried in a jacket pocket, but where did I put it when wearing a summer dress which had no pockets? A flimsy cotton belt was no answer. I did try clipping it to my bra, but that gave me a weird shape as well as being uncomfortable.

The problem brought back memories of coping with the microphone and transmitter for the phonic ear needed by a profoundly deaf pupil. The biggest headache then was not wearing light clothes but thick jumpers. The microphone clip would not take double knitting woollens. As my classroom was virtually circular with no insulation in the flat roof and ill-fitting windows all round, thick clothing was a necessity. I had learnt to adapt, and did likewise with the pager. One easy solution when working at the disabled club was to give my pager to Joan to carry; she always wore jeans so a pocket was available. Joan used to say, "If this bleeper goes off in my pocket, I will have a heart attack, and people will think it's me who must be rushed off, not you."

I remember having the pager clipped to the neckline of a dress and a young girl noticed it and said, "What's that for? Is it a secret camera?"

"No," I replied, "It's like a telephone – if it makes a noise, I know the hospital wants me."

"Oh, are you a doctor or something?"

"That's right," I answered. Of course it did 'make a noise' one evening. I panicked and called to Alan who was in the garden, asking what should I do? I phoned the ward at the hospital in Leeds and was told that I was not required, but had I checked the pager to see if a new battery was needed? Naturally I had not, and naturally a new battery *was* needed.

I decided then that I should read the instructions properly which had been provided with the pager.

Another time I was in the hairdresser's halfway through having my hair trimmed, when there was a continuous bleeping noise. I half jumped out of the chair before I realised that the noise was coming from a new-fangled hairdryer which was in use nearby.

Normally the pager went into my shopping basket or handbag. I had visions of scrabbling amongst the bits of shopping trying to find the pager if it bleeped.

On July 17th my father died. I phoned Leeds to ask if I could go to his funeral in Blundeston. I was not exactly refused permission but was told, "Supposing a heart becomes available; you won't be able to get to Leeds in time." I had previously been informed that I needed to be in Leeds in under four hours if the call came. As Alan said, "You can't do anything for your father and he would not want you to risk it. Cissie has support from her family." This was true. Cissie, my stepmother, or second mother as I preferred to call her, had a son and two daughters, so she would not be on her own, and she understood the problem.

We had told Cissie the transplant news when we had last visited her and my father at the end of March. We did not tell him, as he eighty-eight, and having his first ever spell in hospital. On visiting him, I naturally asked how he was.

He had asked, "How are you?"

"I'm fine," I replied.

He just looked at me with his piercing bright blue eyes and said, "You're a bloody little liar."

We had arranged that if we had any news, we would phone David my stepbrother, and he would inform Cissie. She would then decide if and what to tell my father.

After his death, Cissie said, "Your dad knew that there was something seriously wrong with you. He sensed it."

At the time of his funeral, I decided to walk to the village and sit in the church for a while. I couldn't – the church was locked. This upset me for a few minutes and I remembered something Dad had said. He did not go to church very often. He had worked all his life on the land. He said that he only had to look at a freshly ploughed field with its flock of attendant seagulls, and then see the same field a few months later full of golden waving corn, to appreciate and worship the nature of God. On my way back home I looked with new eyes at the trees surrounding the recreation ground and the flowers and shrubs in our own garden.

I had sent a reading to Cissie which I would have liked to have read out had I been to the funeral. It was read by the minister and I heard afterwards that several people had asked for a copy. I also heard that some people thought me uncaring not to attend my father's funeral. They didn't know the reason.

The reading was written by Henry Scott Holland:

> Death is nothing at all. . . I have only slipped away into the next room. I am I, you are you. Whatever we were to each other that we are still. Call me by my old familiar name, speak to me in the easy way which you always used. Put no difference in your tone, wear no forced air of solemnity or sorrow. Laugh as we always laughed at the little jokes we enjoyed together. Nay smile, think of me, pray for me. Let my name be ever the household word that it always was. Let it be spoken without effort, without the ghost of a shadow on it. Life means all that it ever meant. It is the same as it ever was, there is absolutely unbroken continuity. Why should I be out of mind because I am out of sight? I am waiting for you for an interval, somewhere very near, just round the corner. All is well!

All this time I was ticking off the weeks of waiting. At first every time the phone rang I wondered, 'Is this it?' In the evenings I would not answer the phone, leaving it to Alan – this was cowardly, I know.

In case Alan was not around to take me to Leeds if and when I was needed, the school very kindly offered a number of drivers to get me to the hospital on time. One of the most likely of the drivers was soon unable to oblige. She had broken her ankle badly and was unable to walk, let alone drive a car. I spent many a warm, sunny afternoon with Hazel; we were company for each other. As the end of the school term approached, I knew that the volunteer would not be available so I phoned the ambulance service and was reassuringly told, "Don't worry, love, we'll get you there in time."

I repeated to myself the surgeon's words concerning the length of waiting, 'Two days, two weeks, two months!' If he had continued with 'two years', I would not have bothered, but the two months was over and I had heard nothing.

To make matters worse I was told by a 'friend' who had had a triple-bypass operation himself that if a younger man with a family to support needed a heart and he had the same blood group as you, it was obvious that the heart would go to him. He also implied that at fifty-seven years old I was too old and had had my life. I tried to ignore this, but the niggle remained.

I started to have problems sleeping, or to be more exact staying asleep. I would go to bed at about eleven o'clock and read a bit before sleeping, as I had done for years. Then I would wake at about two o'clock in the morning and that was that; therefore I would be tired during the following day. I knew the time the milkman came to the neighbour's house and heard the goods train which went through at five in the morning. The church clock chimed every quarter as well as the hour. The birds' dawn chorus was very welcome.

Not wanting to rely on sleeping pills, I asked the doctor for his suggestion. "A tot of whisky" was the answer. As I do not like whisky, brandy was substituted.

After consuming a whole bottle of brandy in nightly tots and not sleeping any better, I had to resort to sleeping pills. I only used them every third night to ensure that I got a night's sleep.

Apart from periodic visits to the chest clinic in Halifax and having drugs adjusted, I had no further medical attention. I did go for a cervical cancer smear, which I found quite amusing.

The nurse said, "Before I do the test I'm going to talk about diet. You must eat sensibly so as to take care of your heart—"

I interrupted saying, "Have you read my medical notes?" I could see the notes on the desk.

"No," she replied, "I'll read them afterwards. Now, about looking after your heart—"

"Please read my notes," I pleaded.

"I've told you, I'll read them *afterwards.*"

"But I'm waiting for a heart transplant," I said.

"Oh, well, yes, um – in that case, I'll do your smear!"

In our local daily newspaper at this time were published various articles about a Calderdale man who had had a successful heart transplant and who was busy raising money for the *Yorkshire Evening Post*'s 'Have a heart appeal'. The Government had designated Sheffield as the Regional Transplant Centre, so money was not available under the NHS for Leeds hospitals. As both the General Infirmary and Killingbeck Hospital in Leeds had already performed a number of successful transplants, the *Yorkshire Evening Post* newspaper decided to start an appeal to enable transplantation to continue. Colin's transplant operation had been paid for by this appeal, and he wanted to raise the money which his operation had cost so that someone else would benefit.

Colin was having a 'Fun Day' for his appeal at his local pub, so I went. It was a glorious summer's day and there were many money-raising events and stalls there. If I had not previously seen Colin's photograph in the newspaper, I would never had guessed that he was the one who'd had a transplant a few weeks before. He looked so well and was full of boundless energy and enthusiasm. What a confidence booster he was to me. How good he was at encouraging others to help in his fund raising. I came home feeling so much better for having met him.

The weeks were passing and I was having problems once again with fluid retention. My weight was increasing with the excess fluid. I was a stone heavier than was normal for me. My ankles and feet were so swollen at times that walking became uncomfortable. I found it difficult to eat a large meal as my stomach was becoming distended with the excess fluid. I started using a tea plate instead of a dinner plate for my meals, so I had a plateful of food in front of me.

I still tried to keep active and generally managed to do the weekly shopping, attend the disabled club, visit Hazel whose ankle was taking a long time to heal, entertain friends and family and spend a day at the local gala, though admittedly, I did not work at my usual catering stall in the afternoon.

I was asked to attend another medical tribunal in Huddersfield. My doctor suggested that I should write saying that I was not well enough to attend. He also said that I should contact Leeds General Infirmary as I was obviously deteriorating in health. Another suggestion was to apply for a mobility allowance. I was not at all hopeful about the latter as I had not been granted a disability allowance.

Letters were still coming in frequently from the commissioner's office in London. I remember one letter I wrote after I had been put on the transplant list, asking what I had to do to qualify for a disability allowance – die? I actually tore up one of the letters I received from London because I thought, 'Why bother?' I immediately regretted this and pieced together the letter again with sellotape, because I was fighting for a principle. I also sought help from our solicitor.

One morning he phoned to ask if I had a letter from the commissioner's office, and when I replied in the affirmative he asked, "Can you understand it?"

"No" I answered.

"Neither can I," he replied. "Can you come into the office and I will phone the commissioner's office in your presence!"

I had had to resort to looking up words in the dictionary. Talk about gobbledegook! I thought I had a reasonable understanding of the English language, so it was some comfort to know that a solicitor was having problems, particularly as the legal profession is not renowned for its plain language. We found that the letter implied that my appeal was still being processed.

It was four months since I had been put on the 'list', so I finally contacted the hospital asking for an appointment to see the surgeon.

His secretary said, "But you've been coming to the cardiology unit to see the consultant there." When I said that I had not been to Leeds since just after the assessment, she immediately said, "In that case, you must come to the surgeon's next clinic. I'll fit you in!"

Alan duly took me to Leeds and we had the usual nightmare trying to find somewhere to park. While he was doing that, I wended my way to the waiting area only to find it crowded. I dreaded to think how long I would wait to be fitted in. There was not a vacant seat anywhere. It is thoughtless of people accompanying a patient to take up seats, I thought as I propped myself up against a wall. If I grew tired, I could always slide down and sit on the floor.

The surgeon always came to the door of his office to ask for the next patient. He saw me standing and smiled, at least he had recognised me. To my delight, when he asked for the next patient, it was me! By this time Alan had arrived, so we went in together to see the surgeon.

I was reassured to be told that I had not been forgotten and that I was the only one of my blood group still waiting. However, the surgeon was not happy about the general state of my health and said that he wanted me admitted for drug monitoring. He phoned the cardiac ward and I was admitted. We had had the foresight to pack a bag just in case I was kept in. A bag had been partially packed, ready and waiting, for the last four months. While Alan went to collect my bag, I was taken by wheelchair to Ward 7.

I had to wait outside the ward for some time until a patient due to be released had vacated her bed. There was a rapid turnover of patients on that ward as I soon discovered.

It was back to a single-sex ward. Ward 7 is divided into four rooms with only the eight-bedded coronary care room being mixed; two more rooms had eight beds for either male or female patients, with another room taking the overflow of men.

After being formally admitted and having the usual details written down and an examination by a young house doctor, I was left to inspect my companions.

The atmosphere was friendly and I soon discovered that the lady in the next bed was also called June, and as her surname was Marsden, which was the name of Alan's home village, we soon began chatting. June lived in Leeds and had eight grown-up children, so she always had plenty of visitors and I often benefited from her overflow. June and I still keep in touch with each other. Visiting was allowed from eleven o'clock in the morning until eight o'clock at night, which was very different from the cardiothoracic ward, or the hospital in Halifax.

After numerous tests the following day and visits from the consultant and registrar, pills were readjusted and I was allowed home at the weekend. While Alan and I were leaving that Saturday morning we saw Colin again. He was still fundraising, this time a bed push from Leeds to the General Infirmary in Halifax. The bed, an old hospital one, decked out in balloons, looked most uncomfortable and rickety. There was quite a carnival atmosphere and numerous volunteer 'patients' and an excellent back-up team, including a newspaper van. Colin was bustling around and joking with everyone.

It was good to be home again and to sleep in my own bed! In reply to my correspondence concerning my inability to attend a tribunal in Huddersfield, a letter arrived stating that the date of the tribunal had been set and would be at our home on October 16th. Alan arranged to be at home at the stated time, and Jo, the heart-and-lung transplantee, was coming also. It was suggested that a woman should be present, and who better than Jo?

The altered drugs did not appear to be having any beneficial effect. Many everyday activities were becoming increasingly difficult to do.

Walking to the village, only a few hundred yards, was impossible. For some time the walk down was fine but I found the return up the slight incline difficult. I used to stop frequently and peer into my basket or handbag as if searching for something, stop and take an imaginary stone out of my shoe; fumble in a pocket for a handkerchief and look at children playing or dogs running about on the recreation ground – all subterfuge for needing a chance to catch my breath. I even had to resort occasionally to sitting on the low wall bordering the path and hoping that no one would stop and talk to me as I had no breath left to reply to anyone.

I was fast losing my independence. I had to rely on Alan to take me shopping by car, going from door to door, which was quite a problem sometimes with double yellow lines and narrow roads. Visits to places like the library, doctor, hairdresser and so on had to be made when Alan was available. Necessary ironing was done regularly by a friend with as much as possible just smoothed out and folded. Gladys also called nearly everyday to see if I needed anything to be done or bought.

I had managed to bring in most of the geraniums and fuschias to winter in the greenhouse and to take some cuttings. I had planted some bulbs in pots outside but the greenhouse had to forego its autumn clear out.

Removing the summer bedding plants and setting out pansies and polyanthus for spring had to be left for Alan if and when he had time.

For some time, when cooking the evening meal, I had prepared for three people, one meal being plated up and put in the freezer to help Alan when I was away. I did this until I exhausted my supply of plates.

Going upstairs generally took two or three attempts, a stop being needed after every four rises. When getting up in the mornings I used to get washed and dressed, tidy around and collect everything I needed so that I could stay downstairs. Once a week I stayed upstairs longer to do business accounts for Alan and Geoffrey his business partner. They were working together in a landscape gardening capacity. Sometimes these weekly accounts were sorted out in the early hours when I was unable to sleep.

Christmas presents and cards had been bought early, mainly through mail order catalogues which had dropped through the letter box during the summer months. Presents were wrapped, cards written, addressed and stamped, and left ready to be posted later or hand delivered. I had never been prepared so early for Christmas! Christmas puddings and a large fruit cake had been in the freezer for some weeks and a hamper had been ordered, so things were organised for the forthcoming festive season.

The day of the home tribunal arrived. A short time before the doctor was due to arrive there was a phone call which went something like this:

"Good afternoon, Mrs Buckley, this is the DSS in Leeds. I'm afraid you have been messed about. We have received a message from London via Blackpool to say that the doctors will not be coming this afternoon for your home tribunal!"

'Doctors,' I thought, 'that's the first I knew about doctors. I'm sure only one doctor was mentioned in the letter!' "But why?" I asked. "My husband is having time off work, and a friend is coming from Keighley."

"I don't know," came the reply, "I'm just passing on the messages."

"You must know," I said. "There must have been a reason given to you."

"That's all I know. Goodbye, Mrs Buckley."

A few minutes later the examining doctor also telephoned to say that he and another doctor would not be coming. Again, no explanation was given. Fortunately I had enough time to warn Jo, so she did not have a wasted journey.

We were all puzzled as to why the meeting had not taken place but our doctor, on a routine visit, came up with the answer. He asked if I knew the name of the doctor who was supposed to have come. I did. The doctor was the husband of the woman doctor who had just examined and questioned me in Huddersfield! She worked under her maiden name. Why couldn't this simple explanation have been given to me?

Two days later another doctor came to the house to see if I qualified for mobility allowance. I was very apprehensive about this visit because of the attitude of the doctors when applying for disability allowance. What a difference this time. His friendly, quiet manner soon put me at ease. Apart from answering many questions, I was asked to walk to the front door from the kitchen, having my pulse taken before I started and again at the door.

When I asked if he thought that I qualified, he replied, "I should jolly well think that you do."

"But I don't get a disability allowance," I said. I told him about being assessed as sixty-per-cent disabled and how I was still trying to qualify. I asked him how many people gave up the attempt.

"Nearly everyone," he answered. So much for our Welfare State and National Health Service!

Instead of writing yet another letter to the commissioner's office I decided to write to the Halifax Member of Parliament, Alice Mahon, to see if she could do anything for me concerning the appeal. Mrs Mahon had trained as a nurse and was involved in health matters for the opposition. This letter was planned and written during a sleepless night.

Gladys tentatively made a suggestion one day regarding a wheelchair. She said that if I was amenable and one could be borrowed, I would be able to go to places like Meadowhall in Sheffield where wheelchair access was good. I thought this was a great idea and was looking forward to some outings, however, the best laid plans of mice and men. . .

I had gone to an early evening visit at the local surgery and the doctor said that I should be in hospital. While I was there he phoned through to Leeds and arranged that I was to be admitted the following day, twenty-three weeks after I had been placed on the transplant list.

Returning home, I checked my bag to see that I had everything I needed including something to read. Cheryl had left a novel when she had been staying here saying, "You'll like the Wilbur Smith book, Mum." It wasn't until I looked at the title from my hospital bed that I decided that maybe it wasn't a good choice it was called *A Time to Die*.

On November 1st it was back to Leeds and Ward 7 where the now familiar routine questions were asked and tests were carried out. Again, the friendliness of the staff and patients soon had me feeling relaxed. One lady had been in over two weeks and she had a very dry sense of humour. Over the coming months I came to know Helen extremely well. Alice, in the next bed to Helen, had some years previously undergone a double mastectomy and she had two prostheses, which of course she did not wear in bed. When questioned about the shape and size of a prosthesis, Alice bent down to her locker and brought out the article which was then thrown from bed to bed so we could all examine it. I was amazed at the weight more than anything. A certain amount of hilarity ensued, so much so that we received complaints from the men in the adjoining room that they could not hear the television because of the laughing.

Taking cream cakes and non-alcoholic wine around the entire ward the following evening with the late drink, Alice and I discovered that the male patients who had complained about our hilarity were not such a miserable bunch after all. We did not tell them why we were laughing so much. The 'extras' were provided by a nurse who was celebrating her birthday.

November 5th came, and we could hear the noise of fireworks even though we were unable to see a display. We also had a feast of parkin and other goodies brought in by various patients' visitors. Life in hospital was certainly not dull and gloomy.

So far I was fully mobile, but that changed when I was put on an intravenous drip. I could still go to the bathroom by unplugging the drip stand and turning it on to battery-driven. The next day I was put on two drips and was not allowed food or drink, although I can't remember why. I really was bed-bound then, because there was no way that two drip stands could be manoeuvred. One was bad enough, but two were impossible. Drip stands are similar to supermarket trolleys. They have wills of their own, moving in opposite directions to the one you want. They also have a habit of working perfectly well during the day and malfunctioning throughout the night, emitting a constant bleeping noise until someone attends to them. On one such occasion the exasperated nurse strapped my arm to a wooden splint in an attempt to keep my arm still while I was asleep.

This, too, was unsuccessful. Fun and games also occurred when trying to thread the drip wires through sleeves of nightdress and dressing gown. It was much easier for men who could and did go bare-chested.

Alice went home and we all admired her sweater and shapely figure. As she had to come to a clinic weekly we had several visits from her.

One of the intravenous drips was called a long line drip: this went from my arm to my heart. It was obviously a new procedure for the young houseman as he had the instructions propped up at the end of the bed. He was very pleased when the X-ray taken showed the line in the correct place. I was certainly relieved.

When the time came for the line to be taken out, the same young houseman said, "Did you realise that it was the first time I had done that?"

I replied, "Of course: why else would you have kept referring to the instructions at the bottom of the bed?"

I met a fellow patient some time later who had had the same treatment and who said it was a procedure with which the doctor was familiar, having done it on someone else. I was able to say who that someone was!

Two letters arrived with Alan one evening. One from Alice Mahon MP, wishing me well, but stating that there was nothing she could do concerning my appeal for a disability allowance as I was not in her constituency. She suggested that I should write to my MP and that if I received no help from him, to Sir Donald Thompson. She could then take up my case.

Alan wrote this letter on my behalf as I did not feel like writing, mainly because my writing arm was very sore from the injections which had been administered.

The other letter stated that a mobility allowance had been granted and would be backdated to the date when I had applied, sometime in September. It was ironic that I was granted mobility but not disability.

The same evening, a staff nurse and a student nurse came running to my bed with a wheelchair. While one unplugged the drip stands, the other hustled me out of bed into the wheelchair and off to the nurses' station. Cheryl, our elder daughter, in Canada, was phoning and wanted to speak to me. This was a lovely surprise, but Cheryl could not understand that she was speaking to me on the ward phone which was basically for medical staff only.

"In Montreal," she said, "every bed has its own patient phone." Our talk was necessarily kept short but was especially pleasant as it was a Saturday evening. Weekends in hospital can be somewhat dreary and long, as nothing much happens.

Finally I lost both drip stands. How good it was to be able to walk about freely. What a relief not having to try and steer an unwilling or uncooperative drip stand.

I had named them Fred and Freda and decided that the most awkward one was Fred, being male!

November 14th was our wedding anniversary, and on Alan's daily visit he came armed with a beautiful floral arrangement and a bottle of wine. Those on the ward who could, and wished to, imbibed. It was on this day too that I was asked if I would change my bed position with Helen. She was having an operation the next morning and would need oxygen when she had been given her premedication. There was no oxygen point by her bed. I readily agreed. In my opinion her bed was in the best position as it faced the entrance to the room so one could keep track of all the comings and goings, besides being forewarned of impending visits from doctors.

Alan's sixtieth birthday was three days later was Alan's sixtieth birthday, which he assumed would be spent on his own. Unbeknown to him, it had been arranged that I could go home for the weekend. Alison and family informed Alan that there was no way in which they could travel north that weekend, and then secretly arranged to call in at Leeds on their way from Oxfordshire and collect me.

To say that Alan was dumbfounded when we descended upon him was putting it mildly. A cake that I had made some months previously, which Alan had assumed was for Christmas, had been iced and decorated by a friend, another Hazel. The decorations referred to Alan's likes and habits such as the piano, high jump stand, ash tray, and a spade. It was a wonderful weekend with Christopher and family also coming for the evening meal, prepared by Alison.

The only sad part was that our old cat, Dennis, was now blind and made her way tentatively around the edges of rooms instead of running about as usual.

On Sunday evening we made our familiar journey back to the hospital. By this time we had made ourselves known to the car park attendant at the casualty entrance, so he always allowed us to park there, moving bollards if necessary.

I heard that Helen had had her operation and all had gone well and that she was recovering on the cardiothoric ward. There were also some new inhabitants to get to know. One was an elderly lady who was having her pacemaker renewed. She was sometimes confused, particularly when she had been to the bathroom during the night. She was apt to return to the wrong room, and once the wrong bed. That time it so happened that another patient had gone to the bathroom and when the elderly lady returned first, she got into the other bed. Someone who was awake alerted the nurse, who escorted the lady back to her own bed. Suddenly there was a shriek from the second lady, as she tried to get into bed her feet touched something furry.

"Help!" she yelled. "There's a cat in my bed!" The elderly lady had not removed her fur slippers when she returned from the bathroom.

My stay in this bed position was short lived, because the day after my return from the home visit I found myself in the coronary care unit.

I had been sitting in my bedside chair enjoying the hot lunchtime soup when I fell forward, luckily into an empty soup bowl! The lunchtime soup was generally very good and very hot. This was the first of three cardiac arrests I suffered over the next twelve hours. I remember very little, but I do have odd floating memories. I became aware sometimes of a young male student nurse kneeling by my side, talking to me and asking me to speak to him. I asked him about this some time afterwards, and he said that he had spent over half an hour talking. So I did not dream or imagine that.

At one point a nurse asked me how to get in contact with Alan as the staff thought that he should be with me. I was able to give the nurse the telephone number of Alan's business partner's home after saying that there was no need for Alan to come. I later learned that the hospital had tried for sometime to contact Alan unsuccessfully. Our home phone went unanswered, likewise the bleeper number. Even the police could not contact Alan. Alan always carried the pager with him after that day. I also have vivid memories of running at great speed along a brightly-lit path towards a beautiful garden, which I could just see through a half opened gate. Suddenly I was pulled back and then I was aware of a scream. I suspect it was me screaming when the electrodes gave my heart an electric shock.

The next memory is of being pushed at great speed, or so it seemed, along the hospital corridors. Everywhere was quiet and dimly lit so I assume it was sometime during the night. A hurriedly dressed doctor went ahead opening doors for the porter who was pushing the trolley. A nurse was by my side, talking quietly. A temporary pacemaker was given to me that night, and my right arm felt weighed down by the external battery.

I repeatedly said that I was cold, and more blankets were piled on my bed. My feet were particularly cold and I was aware of Alan rubbing them, trying to warm them for me.

When I was fully conscious and able to sit up, I was aware of sore ribs and could see two reddish circles on my chest – the results of the doctors work trying to keep me alive and succeeding. As one of the nurses told me later, "It wasn't the clapped out machinery which kept you alive but the skill and care of the doctors!"

The coronary care unit was laid out differently from any other ward I had known. There were banks of equipment in the centre of the room with a nurse always watching the screens which were connected to the monitors at each bed. A doctor was always present. There were eight beds, and at least one bed was kept free in case of an emergency admittance. Because of all the equipment, not all the beds were visible to me. Visiting was strictly limited to two visitors per bed and only for a short time in the afternoon and evening. It seemed unfair to the rest of us when one gentleman had several visitors at his bedside throughout the day.

During the second day in coronary care I was trolley driven to the angio suite again for the permanent pacemaker to be fitted until a donor heart became available. The registrar who normally saw to me did this operation and asked who had done the temporary work. When I told him, he said, "I thought it looked like his needlework!" I was a bit miffed because I could not watch what was going on as I had to keep my head turned to the right. Back in my bed, I was again firmly anchored to a monitor, and the monster, mobile, X-ray machine arrived to see if the pacemaker was accurately placed. Sitting up was still painful for my bruised ribs.

The nursing staff talked amongst themselves about the forthcoming Christmas festivities: deciding which parties they were going to attend, the clothes they hoped to buy, who was going with whom, and cruellest of all, what food they were expecting to buy and consume and the drink they hoped to imbibe. Many times I felt like asking them to talk about something else. All their interest about the forthcoming festivities was akin to mental cruelty, we thought.

At some point a technician came with his computerised equipment to test and adjust the pacemaker. Before he started he said, "Of course, you know that six weeks after you leave hospital, you'll be coming back to the pacemaker clinic."

"Oh, no, I won't," I replied.

"Yes, you will," came the answer, "It's normal procedure."

"But I won't," I started to say, "I'm—"

He cut in with, "Yes, you will!" He started the pantomime routine of, "Oh, yes, you will," "Oh, no, I won't."

Becoming rather exasperated, the technician said, "That's the procedure for a patient with a permanent pacemaker."

"But it is not *permanent*," I emphasised.

"Oh, yes, it is." So the pantomime sequence started all over again.

"It's *temporary*," I said finally, "Until I get my transplant."

"I didn't know that," he answered. "I'll just test the pacemaker now."

I really enjoyed that.

Not being able to watch the fitting of the pacemaker, I was curious to know what it looked like. I asked the registrar and he described and drew the article for me. I suppose the best description is that of an old penny flattened at one side. I was shown an X-ray of the pacemaker in place and could read its serial number. I had assumed that as the pacemaker was fitted just below my left shoulder the wiring would go straight down to my heart. Instead, the wires wended their way across the right side of my chest before turning towards my heart.

The day before I left coronary care, I had a surprise visit from Helen, who was brought by wheelchair to see me. She looked very well and her valve operation had been successful. I looked forward to returning her visit to the cardiothoracic ward once I was mobile again and to keeping in touch with her once she returned to her Wakefield home.

It was almost teatime, five days after being taken to coronary care, when I returned to the ward proper, but in yet another different bed position, a corner bed this time. If I stayed in bed much longer, I thought I would have sampled all the different bed positions. There was no one I recognised. The turnover of patients was extremely rapid. A bed never had time to get cold! However, being with the same people twenty-four hours a day meant that one soon gets acquainted.

Visitors were always welcome and I looked forward to six o'clock every evening when Alan came. The timing of his arrival varied depending on the traffic. Alan worked until about four-thirty each day then rushed home for a shower, coffee and change of clothes. He then had to go through the Halifax teatime traffic, meet Leeds rush hour traffic, then find a parking space before arriving at my bedside. It's not surprising that he often fell asleep in the easy chair by the bed.

Visiting hours for Ward 7 were, as previously mentioned, from eleven o'clock in the morning until eight o'clock in the evening, so there was always much coming and going, particularly for patients who lived locally. Alan often brought one of our friends with him and, on the very rare occasion when he did not come, Geoffrey, Alan's partner, and his wife Gladys drove over to Leeds. This was much appreciated.

The unexpected visitors were always a pleasant surprise. June and Alice often popped in with cream cakes on their clinic appointments. Rita, who had also been a Ward 7 patient and who had named me Dormouse, because of my tendency to sleep right under the bedclothes, came quite regularly during the afternoons. Pat, whom I had met when in hospital in Halifax, used to call in when she had arranged to meet her husband before going to the theatre or opera. Frank, Pat's husband, who worked in Leeds, would sometimes spend his lunch hour visiting me.

One morning I looked up to see a large, bearded, young man, clutching bunches of freesias, staring at me.

Ian, whom I had known for many years, had had to come to Leeds to collect some materials for his work, so while he was in the city he had decided to call in to see me. His mother came too, likewise Brenda, an ex-teaching colleague, and Ronnie, her husband, when they were shopping in Leeds.

Every Sunday afternoon Hazel hobbled along the hospital corridors to my bedside. She was still unable to drive, so her fiancé, Bryan, brought her before he returned to London where he worked during the week. Alan would come on Sundays in the late afternoon, stay for a while, and then go out to get something to eat before returning to the ward. Quite often he went to a McDonalds and brought me back a strawberry milkshake.

Our local GP surprised me one evening by coming in briefly to see how I was faring. Another pleasant surprise was the day visit from Kate, who lived in Essex. We had taught together many years ago and always remained friends. We spent a very enjoyable day. Kate is always amusing.

One morning I heard chattering and laughter coming from the nurses' station and recognised one of the voices as belonging to Colin, the Calderdale transplant. I quickly got out of bed and went to see him. It was a joyful reunion for me and I was introduced to two more of the 'gang', John and Don. Don was the first transplant patient from Leeds General Infirmary, and John had had his transplant two months previously. This meeting really made my day and I returned to my bed feeling somewhat smug. The 'gang' had come for routine blood tests and an examination, plus a general chat with the ward staff. They looked so well and full of the joys of living.

Christmas was approaching and there were the usual once yearly letters to write. I wrote a few each day. It was, for most of the recipients of my letters, the first they knew of my health problem. They were obviously surprised and shocked by the news, judging from the replies I received.

Another tribunal to find out if I qualified for a disability allowance had been arranged to take place in Leeds. I had signed a letter which enabled Alan to represent me as I was not well enough to attend myself. All the time that letters had been to-ing and fro-ing between my home and London, no medical questions or assistance had been requested. The local doctor, cardiologists from Halifax and Leeds, the cardiothoracic surgeon – no one had been contacted to query my case, even though I had obtained permission from all the medics to give their names and addresses. By this time, Cheryl, our lawyer daughter, in Canada, had written or faxed various letters, and Alison in Oxfordshire had contacted medics and the DSS. Alan had written to anyone and everyone he could think of who might have some influence. Sir Donald Thompson had also appealed to the commissioner's office.

It was not until the weekend before the tribunal that the cardiac consultant who was caring for me was approached by the board.

I knew this because Dr Smith asked for my permission to use my medical notes in a letter to the tribunal committee.

Alan was set to wage war at the tribunal, when the wind was completely taken out of him. When he entered the room, the chairman, who had various pieces of paper in front of him, including the consultant's letter, said that the appeal had been granted and would be backdated. However, Alan was not prepared to leave the room without having his say. He proceeded to tell the members of the tribunal exactly what he thought. His parting comment stated that it was not the money we had been fighting for, but the principle.

Hopefully, other people would benefit from our persistence. Alan came straight from the tribunal to tell me the good news and Dr Smith also came to find out the result.

Life on Ward 7 carried on as usual. Monday was the ward cleaning day. Beds, chairs, tables and lockers were moved round to enable the floor to be cleaned and polished. I recall one of these Mondays in particular. It was when I was attached to a machine, so my bed could not be moved. As my locker was on the other side of the room, momentarily, as I looked across, I thought, 'Someone has the same towels as me.' I could see the towels hanging on the rail at the back of the locker. I quickly realised that it was *my* locker, and on the floor nearby were a pair of my panties which had been drying on the locker hook. I called across to the cleaner and asked if she would pick them for me. Her comments were hilarious and she finally said, "I bet it's not the first time you've dropped your knickers."

Whenever I saw her after this, either on the ward or along the corridors, she always addressed me as Mrs Knickers!

I was told regularly that I would probably go home for the weekend, but then for some unknown reason my temperature would rise in the evenings and my hopes would be dashed. Having a fan by my bedside plus most of the bedclothes removed made no difference. Each morning my temperature was acceptable, only to rise drastically in the evening.

I was also retaining a large amount of fluid on my stomach. The diuretic dosage was fairly high and there was some concern that my kidneys might be permanently damaged. My distended stomach meant that eating a full meal became impossible, as after a few mouthfuls I felt bloated and extremely full. Even after receiving the small portions of food I asked for, I still left a great deal. I always felt guilty because, when I was a child, my mother was against the wastage of food. "Think of all the starving children," she would say. "They'd be glad to eat your food." My stomach became so distended that the registrar used to greet me in the mornings with, "How are your quads this morning?"

The rest of my body was becoming thinner. I had given my rings to Alan to take home because I thought I could lose them as they slipped off my fingers so easily.

As I was in a teaching hospital, permission was regularly asked for students to examine patients. I became very familiar with these examinations and was often a step ahead of the students' requests to look at my eyes, tongue, fingernails, and pulse in my neck. On one occasion there were only two students plus a doctor who approached my bed, instead of the usual six or more. Both students seemed extremely nervous, and most of the examination had been completed under the eagle eyes of the doctor. Then she was called away. Immediately one of the students said, "Do you know what's wrong with you?" When I replied in the affirmative, he said, "Go on, please tell us." So I did!

I saw the students again the next day and asked if they had diagnosed me correctly to the doctor.

"Yes," was the answer.

"What did she say?" I queried.

"She said, 'she's told you'," said the student. "We didn't dare deny it either."

One evening when Alan came, we were chatting away in the normal way about everyday matters, when Alan suddenly said, "I wasn't going to tell you, but I've had to have Dennis put down this morning." I didn't say anything for a moment and then started to cry. Very soon Alan joined me, so we drew the bed curtains and both had a good weep. Dennis had had a brain haemorrhage, and as soon as the vet saw her he said that there was nothing he could do. After walking aimlessly around Hebden Bridge for a while, Alan returned to the vet's surgery to collect Dennis' body and bring her home to be buried in one of her favourite spots in the garden.

Dennis was not originally our cat – she had been our elder daughter's. While Cheryl was a student in Exeter, she phoned home one evening to say, "We've found a gorgeous black kitten in the road. No one has claimed it, so we have taken it in. It's a real little menace though, and since it got its head stuck in the marmalade jar, we've called it Dennis the Menace."

A few weeks later a phone call went something like this. "Mum, you know that little kitten? Well, the landlord says we can't keep it. What shall we do?"

"Find it a home," was my answer. So she did. Cheryl and Dennis arrived together for the Christmas vacation. Dennis was wearing a pale blue collar and lead because, "He's male, Mum, the vet said so, and he's house trained!"

We soon discovered that 'he' was not male, and six months later was not house trained. We had had Dennis for over sixteen years. For the first time in our married lives we would be without a cat.

After Alan had left that sad evening, concerned patients asked what had been wrong. Why had we drawn the curtains?

"My cat has died," I wailed.

The same evening a patient came from the cardiothoracic ward. It was Helen. She was having problems with fluid retention and was very poorly. Also, she had received the sad news that her husband had died.

Helen was distraught. She blamed herself for not being at home with him. The nursing staff were wonderful and we all did our utmost to help her and her daughter Jackie, who visited regularly.

I felt like a permanent fixture in the hospital by now, and if a patient wanted to know anything about the running of the ward, someone was bound to say, "Ask June." Patients came and went; no one stayed for more than a few days except Helen and myself.

One foreign lady had her porter son visit her for a few minutes whenever he was nearby. I was asked to plait her long hair for her, but I doubt if I did it to her entire satisfaction.

Another elderly patient was celebrating her seventieth birthday. She was an amusing character. When she had fallen asleep the night before her birthday, the staff festooned the curtain rail above her bed with lavatory paper and made a banner saying, HAPPY BIRTHDAY HANNAH. They found a spare slipper from somewhere and decorated that too. Hannah had mislaid one of her slippers and was forever asking if anyone had found a slipper, size seven.

I was still quite mobile and able to walk about freely. Returning from the bathroom, I used to see a man sitting in a chair by his bed in the room which faced the bathroom corridor. I started to wave as I went along and he used to smile and wave back. Then we began calling out, "Good morning," or whatever was appropriate for that time of day. Finally I decided to go into the three-bedded, male room and chat to him. He was a local Leeds man and we talked about things in general. One evening a new patient was in one of the beds and Harold said, "He's worried sick. I wonder if you would speak to him. He's having a pacemaker fitted tomorrow."

I walked across and became acquainted with Malcolm. I explained about my pacemaker. I think I eased his worries. The next day Malcolm was trolleyed off and returned cheerfully having had his operation. Going for my regular evening chat with Harold, we overheard a conversation between Malcolm and his wife and daughters. We almost made ourselves ill with suppressed laughter. Malcolm's family were asking about his operation, how he felt, and what he needed bringing in on their next visit. Malcolm's request baffled them. He asked for a watch chain. When they asked, "What for?", he replied, "To attach to my pacemaker, so that when I go to the local pub I can pull out the pacemaker and show it to my mates." He kept his face absolutely straight, and for a while his family believed him. It was Harold's and my laughter which made them suspicious and realise that Malcolm was having them on!

Malcolm then requested more pyjamas. His family certainly got their revenge. When they arrived the next day, they hastily bundled up his other pyjamas before presenting him with a new pair. They had a large Mickey Mouse pattern all over them.

Towards the end of visiting one evening, a woman came to see me and asked where my operation would take place. I said, "Here in Leeds. Why?"

She replied, "I've just come from visiting my husband in coronary care. He needs a heart transplant but has been told that he will have to go to Newcastle for the operation."

"Why?" I asked.

"Because Leeds have no money," was the answer. "Are you sure your operation will be here in the Infirmary?"

"As far as I know," I replied. Nevertheless I thought about her news and there was a niggle in my mind on and off all night. I eagerly awaited the registrar's morning visit. As usual, he answered my query in his quiet friendly, straightforward manner and said, "Why, here of course."

"But Leeds haven't any money for such things, so I've been told," I said.

"We have money for *your* operation," was the reassuring reply.

When I asked how the would-be heart transplant patient was faring, I was told that he hadn't made it – in other words, he had died.

I then overheard the nursing staff talking about Mr Murday, the transplant surgeon, who had decided to leave because of the lack of funding for transplants. He was going to St George's Hospital in London where transplants could be performed. I learned that the Government had designated Sheffield, not Leeds, as the Transplant Centre for Yorkshire. Money would therefore be allocated to Sheffield for these operations.

On asking what would happen to me if I had not had my new heart before the surgeon left, I was told, "Oh, you'll go to London attached to him." I had visions of running along the M1 holding on to a piece of string!

"How will I get to London?" I asked.

"Either in an ambulance with a police escort, or perhaps by helicopter."

I must admit that I did not fancy that at all, and just hoped that the surgeon was still in Leeds when a donor organ became available.

Now patients *do* have to go to London from Leeds hospitals for their transplants. It's a long distance from home and expensive for visitors and follow-up examinations. It was almost Christmas and I pleaded to be allowed home. Nearly every day I was told, "Maybe tomorrow." There is the saying that 'tomorrow never comes' – it certainly felt like it to me.

Finally the news came. I could have Christmas leave even if my temperature was still high. On the morning of December 21st Alan came for me and home I went. My joy was short-lived though, as by the evening of the 22nd I was breathless and not feeling very well. Alan phoned the hospital and by ten o'clock I was back again in Leeds. My bed was still available as admissions, except for emergencies, had been suspended because of the Christmas period. There were only three of the eight beds occupied, one by Helen who was showing very little improvement.

After a late night X-ray and examination I was given an extra large diuretic dose, so I had precious little sleep that night. However, after another day, when the room was almost denuded of patients I was told that I could go home for a few days. I was asked to keep a chart of my temperature both morning and night, and told to sit and do nothing except get bored.

We could have a very quiet, unfestive Christmas Day, I thought. In the morning we opened our presents, which were under the Christmas tree as usual. Alan had brought in, planted, and decorated a Christmas tree for my return home, and he had also put up some coloured lights outside the house – a new venture for us! Hazel had asked us to join her family for an evening meal which we enjoyed. We did not stay for long and had returned home when Alison phoned, she said, "We have had our Christmas Day, the children are fast asleep in bed, and Tony and I are just sitting here looking at television. Would it be all right if we came now instead of the morning?"

Alison had originally arranged to come to Yorkshire on Boxing Day for a few days, to cook for us and see us. When she knew that I would be home for Christmas, she had arranged the visit north but I had said that she should have Christmas Day at home with the children first.

"Of course you can come now," we said. The family with two sleepy children arrived before midnight. I reckoned that it was exactly thirty-one weeks since I had been put on the transplant list.

I was expected back in Leeds on the evening of December 27th. It was very wet and windy and Alison asked how I felt. Would I prefer to travel during the day, she asked. Naturally, I wanted another evening with the family and my own bed. The hospital gave permission for me to delay my return until midday on the 28th. I felt like Cinderella.

As we were driving from the house the following morning just before eleven o'clock, I said to Alan, "I haven't got my pager."

"You won't need it," said Alan, "Especially as we're on our way to Leeds."

At ten minutes past eleven, staff at the hospital tried to contact me to say that a suitable heart might be available. Alison took the call and immediately telephoned Cheryl and Christopher to tell them the news. She also contacted some friends. Alan and I, of course, knew nothing until we reached the ward just before midday.

Immediately nurses came running up, laughing and saying, "We've some great news."

"What is it?" I asked. "Am I going home again?"

"Much better than that – it's a heart."

What wonderful, somewhat unbelievable news! I was excited and so were the nurses who continued smiling and laughing as I clambered out of the wheelchair which I had used from the casualty entrance to the ward. Everyone in sight was cuddled. Alan looked worried and apprehensive. It was far worse for him as a spectator.

There were some strange faces in the ward beds which had once again been filled. Helen was there in her usual corner bed. I went across and chatted excitedly to her. She was looking rather better and not so bloated with fluid. She told me about the Christmas festivities which had taken place for the depleted number of patients on the ward.

One of the new patients said, "So *you're* June. Every time someone comes into the room there is the comment, 'Oh, that's June's bed!' Now I know who June is!"

Alan and I sat on the bed talking, about what I have no idea. It was not long before a young houseman came up and put a damper on my high spirits.

He said, "It may not happen. We don't know yet if the heart is suitable."

Mr Murday bustled in and told us that it would be about three hours before they would knew if the donor organ was compatible. He said that I should have nothing to eat or drink just in case the operation was performed. I had had one small slice of toast and marmalade and a cup of coffee that morning, but I was too excited to feel hungry. I suggested to Alan to go to the canteen for a drink at least, but I honestly cannot remember if he had anything or not.

I looked at the ward clock to estimate at what time I would be certain that it would happen. I then tried not to look at the clock too often.

It was a very long afternoon, but nurses continued to come and talk to me. A lovely floral arrangement arrived from Alison and family wishing me luck. The anaesthetist came and sat on my bed, asking various questions and explaining the procedure he would be carrying out if. . .

At some point Alan must have left the ward as he could not have gone so long without a cup of coffee, or more importantly, a cigarette. We were told that a 'harvesting' team had gone to Hull to collect organs from the donor. This seemed an odd word to use but we could not think of another way to describe this action.

The magical three hours had passed, then four hours. At this point I merely shrugged my shoulders and thought, 'Well, it's not going to happen today, but I know that something will happen sometime!'

One of the nurses came in briskly, saying, "Have you had a bath yet?"

"No, why?" I asked.

"Come on, quickly, you need to bathe and put on your gown. I'll go and run the bath. It's nearly time for your pre-med!"

"Is it going ahead then?"

"As far as we know. Once you're in the bath, I'll change your bed position so that you can have oxygen!"

I duly had my bath and donned the white operating gown. When I returned, my bed had been moved. I was given a pre-med dosage and an oxygen mask. I asked if the latter was necessary and was told emphatically that it was. It was not so easy trying to talk with a mask covering the nose and mouth.

The same nurse, Julie, materialised again and said that she would come with me and Alan to the operating theatre. A porter and trolley appeared, and I was wheeled out of the ward with everyone calling out, "Good Luck. See you soon."

Alan and Julie came as far as the door of a small room and there they left me to the anaesthetist. The surgeon had said that a room in the hospital was available for Alan's use that night, but it was decided that he would be happier at home with the family rather than alone in a bleak hospital room. Mr Murday said that he would phone Alan as soon as the operation was over.

The anaesthetist talked all the time he was putting the lines into my left wrist. I found this very painful. He had also said that I could wake up and find that nothing had happened as something might not be suitable at the last minute. I turned my head so that a line could be put into my neck, and that is all I remember.

I had left the ward just before nine o'clock on the evening of December 28th, and at two-thirty the next morning Mr Murday kept his word and phoned home, saying that the operation was over and successful. We have photographs of that joyous moment. What a dreadful time it must have been for those waiting back home.

That afternoon, I am told, Alison and Alan came to see me in the intensive care unit and I had a perfectly normal conversation with Alison. Alison was the only visitor allowed. She was returning with her family to Oxfordshire later that afternoon, so Alan stayed outside the glass-panelled door.

Apparently, I waved to Alan and asked him to bring me my glasses from the ward. I also reminded him to water the house plants back home. I remember nothing of this.

Life After the Operation

My first memory of waking up was seeing a nurse sitting at a table in a pool of light, while the rest of the room appeared to be dark. I was in a half-sitting position, and looking down I saw what can best be described as a spaghetti-like mass of wires. I immediately thought that something had happened.

I called across to the nurse and asked her the time.

"Two o'clock," was the answer. "How do you feel?"

"Fine," I replied, and I did. I was so relieved to be able to speak.

The only thing which had concerned me, or worried me, about the whole operation was being on a ventilator with a tube down my throat and not being able to talk. I learned later that I had only needed a ventilator to help my breathing for about four hours after the operation.

The nurse had said, "Two o'clock," but I didn't know whether it was early morning or afternoon, as the intensive care unit was underground. Everywhere was very quiet. Did that mean it was night or because it was the intensive care area? As it was some time before Alan came to visit, I assume that it was two o'clock in the morning when I woke up.

I was surprised to feel no pain and to feel so well. I was given a sickly sweet drink, and the machines to which I was attached were regularly checked. The diabetes testing 'clothes peg' on the finger amused me. I found it much preferable, however, to the finger pricking which was carried out for some days later on.

I was helped out of bed into a chair, where I sat for nearly three hours. Alan was very surprised at that when he eventually came to visit me, gloved and aproned.

A nurse was always with me in the room and no one else was allowed in apart from doctors and physiotherapists. Everyone had to thoroughly wash their hands before entering. The bed was extremely comfortable as it could be cranked into various positions, but the bed linen was a different matter. Everything was sterile, from sheets and nightdresses to towels and flannels. Using a towel was akin to rubbing my face on rough emery paper! The nightdress came out of a sterile packet, like a piece of cardboard. It also had Velcro on the shoulders, enabling easy changing and avoiding having to thread wires through sleeves.

During the following days a number of wires were disconnected from the wrist line. The end of the line reminded me of the head of a violin with a number of knobs, which on a violin could tighten or loosen the strings. I was also attached to an external pacemaker, the box of which was fixed over the end of the bed. I was out of bed in the chair for five hours that day. When Alan came, he said that he had been busy answering the phone and making phone calls. There was still no feeling of pain, and apart from feeling drowsy, I was well.

It was shortly after midnight and I was more or less asleep, when the 'resident' nurse said quietly, "June, there's someone to see you. Are you awake enough?" The house doctor and the nurse had come from Ward 7 to wish me a Happy New Year. It was now 1991. A New Year and the start of my new life.

The doctor had started on the ward the day I was admitted, on November 1st. He had also put in my long line: his first, as previously mentioned. I had seen him on his long weekend stint getting more and more weary. He was always ready to attend to a patient though, and as Ward 7 was a cardiac ward, there was always someone who needed attention. I felt as though I knew him quite well.

I was expected to leave intensive care on that day, but it was decided that another day would be more beneficial. As it was a bank holiday, it was not certain that the cleaning staff would be available to clean my room on the Cardiothoracic Ward. A routine had been established of me sitting in the chair, doing breathing exercises, having machines checked, and talking to whichever nurse was on duty.

I was definitely going to Ward 23 on the following day, January 2nd. It was later than expected, as I had to wait until another X-ray had been taken. Finally I was on my way, still in my comfortable bed. I was taken quickly through the corridors and lifts to a small room near the entrance to Ward 23.

My primary nurse came in, took one look at me, and said, "I know you."

I looked at him and said, "I know you."

Martin had been on the nursing staff of the ward in Halifax which I had got to know so well, and he had recently transferred to Leeds.

I was told that I would have no visitors apart from Alan, who would have to wash thoroughly before coming in and leave his outdoor clothing outside the room. The nursing staff also had to wash their hands every time they re-entered the room. Martin's hands soon began to look red and sore. I could not have any flowers, newspapers, handle money, or have a library book because of the risk of infection. On my bed, though, when I arrived at the ward, was my first 'Get Well' card. It was from Colin, who had been in for a biopsy but could not wait to see me because of the metered car parking. The card welcomed me to the 'gang'.

When the room door opened, I could see that there were notices pinned on the outside which said, NO VISITORS, HANDWASHING AND APRONS NECESSARY, NO ADMITTANCE, SEE SISTER. I felt like adding another one, DANGEROUS ANIMAL. There was a round porthole window in the door, and as the room was at the beginning of the ward visitors and anyone leaving had to pass my door. As walking patients were going past with their visitors I would hear comments such as, "The transplant is in there!" Faces would appear through the porthole window. I felt rather like a freak – Frankenstein came to my mind.

My comfortable bed was taken away and I was issued with one of the normal hospital variety. I didn't sleep very well. I had forgotten how noisy the ward could be after the solitude of the Intensive Care Unit. I still had a nurse with me full-time. Martin was in whenever it was his shift. Nel, who was shortly getting married, was also a regular. She talked about her forthcoming wedding arrangements, which certainly helped to pass the time.

Martin was very strict, and I could not get away with anything. I often started to say, "Martin, can I—" or "Martin, would it—" I never got any further because he always butted in with, "No, you can't," or, "No it wouldn't."

I longed for a bath and to wash my hair, but. . . The window blind was temperamental and at my request Martin fixed it so that it stayed up. I could then see the sky and watch the clouds skidding by. On Ward 7 the view from the windows was very uninspiring – a red brick wall.

The day after becoming a resident of Room 2 on Ward 23 I was taken for a walk with Martin. We walked along the corridor, away from the ward, towards the empty dayroom. I was masked, and Martin carried my pacemaker machine. This was surprisingly heavy, it looked similar to a large transistor radio. My legs felt somewhat wobbly but it felt good to be mobile again.

During that afternoon a reporter and a photographer from the *Yorkshire Evening Post* came. The surgeon had come in earlier. He had sat on my bed and asked if I would talk to the press. I said that I would rather not. Mr Murday then suggested that I talked it over with Alan.

I asked, "Will it help in any way?"

"Yes," was the reply. "It will bring in money, and maybe a donor."

I had waited seven months for a donor, so if someone else could forego such a wait I was prepared to talk to anyone. Therefore I said, "Yes, I don't need to talk it over with Alan."

Within a short space of time, or so it seemed to me, the reporter arrived. It was then that I realised that my operation had not been paid for by the National Health but by the appeal organised by the *Yorkshire Evening Post*. Their 'Have a Heart' appeal had been started to enable transplants to be continued in Leeds after the government had stopped funding such operations. It would have been churlish not to speak to the press. Photographs were taken with Martin by my side.

So began the press coverage. There had already been snippets in the Halifax daily newspaper, the *Evening Courier*. Another Calderdale person had benefited from the same donor. He had had a single lung operation in a Bradford hospital. He also was recovering well.

Our local weekly newspaper commented at length, mostly correctly. When a friend went into a newsagents on this publication morning, a customer remarked aloud on the transplant headline in large print on the front page. "Just fancy, a local woman has had a heart transplant."

Joan replied, "Yes, she's a friend of mine! The woman then said, "Goodness me, I've never met anyone who knows someone who's had a heart transplant."

I did not get to read the press articles for a few days, as I was still not allowed newspapers or flowers. I did receive mail though, which seemed rather odd. Surely that would be as 'dirty' as newspapers? The press reporter and photographer had been in with their equipment. I believe that they had to wash their hands.

I was asked if I would like a television, so one was brought in, having first been well washed with disinfectant. Feeling somewhat apprehensive about switching on the set because of its watering, I pretended that I didn't know where the controls were, so I asked a nurse. The black and white set worked well enough.

I was only allowed hot food, no salads or fruit. I regularly had a tin of soup for a meal, as who needs two hot, cooked meals a day? A carton of yoghurt was my dessert at every meal.

The day following my first walk, I went with a physiotherapist for two further walks, including going down and then up a short flight of stairs – five in number. My thigh muscles protested strongly.

Earlier that day, while it was still dark, I had been awakened by an almighty crash.

The wind had blown open my window, sending bottles, pills, and other paraphernalia which had been on the window sill tumbling everywhere. I tried shutting the window but the wind was too strong. I shouted, "Help," at the top of my voice. A nurse came running followed by two others, and after a struggle the window was closed. I started thinking then about the boxes of drugs back on the window sill. Surely they should have been locked away? I went back to sleep in spite of the howling gale.

Some restrictions were lifted and I was able to have flowers in my room and to display the growing number of 'Get well' cards. My room did not feel or look so barren. I was told that I was to be in Room 2 for at least three weeks. I could cover the wall with cards and put flowers anywhere I wanted. I asked Alan to bring in photographs of our children, grandchildren, or home and garden. Those I arranged on a large sheet of card and placed near my bed and easy chair so that I could look at them.

Every evening Alan brought in that day's cards, and I enjoyed arranging them after visiting hours. One was different from the others. It stated, 'On your achievement.' It certainly was an achievement to survive as I had done. I was amazed at the number of cards I received and from whom. The grapevine had certainly spread its tendrils.

Saturday and Sunday were relatively quiet, but not so much as on Ward 7. The surgeon still made his twice daily visits, often in tracksuit and trainers instead of suit or operating garb. Physiotherapy continued and a pair of pedals was brought in so that I could start to strengthen my leg muscles. My pulse was taken before I started pedalling, and again after a minute. When I enquired why, I was told that as the nerves to my heart had been severed I would not know when I had done too much. This was something I had not realised. I suppose that was the reason why I had had no chest pains.

I was taking regular doses of the anti-rejection drug, so far in a liquid form. This was very syrupy, so the easiest way was to syringe it into my mouth. Martin took delight in telling me about the size of the anti-rejection pill I would soon be taking. (Although quite large, shaped like the liquorice torpedo sweet, it did slip down easily.) I also had steroid pills at regular intervals and began to develop a familiar 'moon' face. Alan called me Hamster Features.

Martin was not on duty that first weekend and the nurse who called for me was wonderful, so motherly. I was able to have my hair washed in the wash basin in my room, and on Sunday morning I was taken for a bath, for which I had pleaded. I certainly relished that, in spite of the fact that the bathroom was unheated. It was great being pampered. I thought: 'I could get used to this.'

On Martin's return on Monday morning, I mentioned my weekend activities, to which he simply replied, "I've heard." Before nine o'clock that Monday morning I was once again travelling along the corridors for a biopsy on my new heart. This meant an hour and a half lying flat on my back when I returned to my room, then a complete spell of sitting up in bed before being allowed to get up later in the afternoon.

The biopsy results were satisfactory, so there was no need to be 'special' nursed anymore. My room door was open and I was allowed to mingle with the other patients. I could also get dressed during the day. I felt human once again.

The day after the biopsy, I met another transplant patient who was in for a routine biopsy. John was a great character and I spent most of the morning talking to him. The following morning, Ken, Don and another John all appeared on the ward for their regular blood tests for Cyclosporin (the anti-rejection drug) levels. There was much chatting, joking, and merriment.

As Alan was leaving that evening, he took me by wheelchair to Ward 7 so that I could see the nursing staff I had got to know so well, and especially to visit Helen. I was made very welcome and thoroughly enjoyed the sense of freedom. A nurse took me back to my room.

Unfortunately, Colin was back in hospital, in the room adjacent to mine, but no one was allowed in his room except the medical staff, of which there was a continual stream. After a while, Colin was taken to the intensive care unit. I had a quick chat to him before he was whisked away. However often I asked, I could get no further news of Colin.

On the morning of January 10th, I seemed to have a number of visits from the nursing staff, mostly just popping in to say hello. They all avoided my queries regarding Colin. Later in the morning Colin's wife came in to tell me that Colin had died. I thought it was so brave of her to come herself to tell me. Colin had been a larger than life character and a wonderful confidence-booster to me. His wife said that almost Colin's last words were, "Tell June to fight and fight and fight. It won't happen to her!"

Everyone was subdued, and the nursing staff continued to call in at my room throughout that sad day. Mr Murday's words were both comforting and reassuring, repeating Colin's words that it wouldn't happen to me!

The ward staff were going to a 60s disco the next evening, and I had previously overheard them wondering and discussing what to wear. I had given a note to Alan to take to Gladys, asking her to look through my wardrobe and bag up anything which might be suitable for a 60s theme.

As my daughters tell me that I never throw anything away, I felt confident that Gladys would find some suitable articles of clothing. On the morning of Colin's death a number of plastic bags containing clothing were piled up against the wall in Room 2 for nurses to rummage through. It certainly helped that day along.

On the evening of the disco the ward staff came along dressed in their 60s gear. They certainly looked different, and I for one had difficulty in recognising some of them. They said afterwards that they had a good time. The certainly deserved it.

It was decided that it was about time that my room was cleaned. I was asked to stand outside so that I would not inhale dust. As I was standing in the corridor, looking at the photographs displayed on the wall, the anaesthetist came by and stopped to chat. After a few minutes he said, "You're a lot more talkative today than you were on the night of the operation!"

"Did I say anything?" I asked.

"No," he said. "I kept saying, 'Speak to me, June' but you wouldn't."

"Are you sure?" I queried, as I knew that people can say the oddest things when under an anaesthetic. I was relieved when the anaesthetist replied, "I couldn't get a word out of you."

I just hope that was true!

One of the ward sisters had returned from a few days leave and she told me that she had watched my operation, although she had found it hard to keep awake. She had been on duty all day and was then in the theatre until the early hours of the next morning. She said that she had helped with the saline bags. I asked her if she had seen my lungs.

"Yes," she replied, sounding somewhat puzzled.

"What colour were they?" I asked.

"Pink, why?" was the reply. "You don't smoke, do you?"

"No, but I live with a very heavy smoker," I said, "So I expected my lungs to be black."

"I can assure you they were not black."

This was a relief, as we hear so much about passive smoking nowadays.

Every day, more flowers arrived, and I spent time every morning watering and rearranging where necessary. Fresh flowers have a limited life in the dry, centrally heated atmosphere in hospital. I wrote many letters of thanks and replies to letters received. Knitting a 'Spot the dog' jumper for Rhiannon, our granddaughter and reading took up more time. Probably the most time was spent just chatting to other patients and friends who came visiting. I made regular trips to Ward 7, on my own two legs, mainly to see Helen who was thankfully getting better. She had been moved nearer the ward entrance, so, we said, the next move would be out altogether.

The Church of England chaplain for the hospital came round regularly during the week as well as holding ward communion services on Sundays.

One day she called into my room and asked me how I felt now that the transplant was over.

"Very humble," I said. "Why should so much money be spent on me? Why should *I* be given a second chance?" Her reply was that I could show my thanks by getting fully better and staying that way. This did not answer my queries, but it made me more determined than ever to live a normal life once again.

Every afternoon after lunch, which was approximately at midday, we were supposed to be in bed and to have a rest. This was known as the 'Happy Hour'. I generally went to sleep in spite of the noise from the nearby kitchen and the chattering of the nurses. I was frequently surprised at how quickly the days passed. It is easy to become institutionally orientated when all thinking is arranged for one. Our days were geared to meal times and visiting times, the tea trolley and the pill trolley, doctors' visits and temperature taking, early rising and bedtime.

On the Sunday morning, two weeks after my transplant, there were numerous complaints and moans, mostly from the men. The newspaper trolley had not appeared. I heard the sister call out, "We're too busy to go for them. Anyone with two legs can go and fetch your newspapers."

There was no reply to this, so after a few minutes I said, "I'll go." I went round the ward, making a list of which paper was needed at which bed and collecting money.

Armed with list and money, I made my way to the newspaper stall situated at the front entrance to the hospital. This involved going down the lift to the ground floor level, walking along a long corridor, and eventually turning into the imposing Victorian entrance. I collected and paid for thirteen newspapers in variety and staggered back to Ward 23. I had forgotten how bulky and heavy Sunday newspapers had become with all their different section and colour supplements. Having delivered the newspapers, I found I had some extra money. Everyone said I had given them their correct change, so somewhere, somehow I had made a profit.

Then the next day, at the start of another week, I went to the gymnasium at last. I had found the pedals rather dull, so I used to read while pedalling. My first short visit to the gym that morning was most disappointing. I was shown the gym and the equipment. Having taught physical education and taken weekly assemblies for years in a gym, I certainly knew what one looked like. After protesting, I was allowed to use the exercise bicycle for two minutes. However, I went back to the gym that same afternoon for a short series of structured exercises. Those were mainly to strengthen my leg muscles, and involved such exercises as sitting down and standing up (without using my arms as leverage), walking up the rungs of the wall bars, and more step climbing. I also used a large ball, not as heavy as a medicine ball, pushing it up into the air when lying flat with my hands. Everything was done in units of five, the aim being to reach a further five at subsequent visits.

Each session ended with a spell on the exercise bicycle. It was somewhat distressing to see that some of the other patients receiving physiotherapy in the gym were young men who had had bad injuries from motor accidents.

Because I was so keen to get back my strength, I was always ready for a visit to the gym, but these visits were erratic as I could only go when a physiotherapist was available to come with me. I was told that I was worse than the patients who were lethargic – I wanted to do too much!

When the *Halifax Courier* reporter and photographer came to visit me, I said that I was not going to be interviewed in bed because I wasn't an invalid. I took them 'along the Victorian corridors of Leeds General Infirmary' – to quote the newspaper – to the gymnasium, where I was photographed on the exercise bicycle. I did not enjoy this, as photograph after photograph was taken.

I watched the television, mainly to hear news about the forthcoming Gulf War. After days of speculation, on January 17th, the Gulf War started. There had been talk of the hospital becoming a centre for head injuries, and to this end the visits to the gymnasium were accompanied by much banging and drilling. The gym was to become a ward. The floor was taped out so that the electricians working from the floor above could see where the beds were to be placed, hoops of wiring hung down everywhere, and equipment was moved around. Medical staff, including physiotherapists, were prepared to leave the hospital for the war front when and if needed, so there was often a subdued and sombre atmosphere around the hospital.

As I had finished the jumper I was knitting, I decided to try my hand at designing a family tree tapestry. Armed with a book of cross-stitch designs, graph paper, pencils, crayons, scissors and erasers, I set to work and spent several hours sorting and planning a design. The nursing staff and patients showed an interest, and I was never short of company as I sat at a table working. When the night staff came on duty, I had to return the table, as it was used by them on the ward. Everyone wanted to see the finished tapestry, but as yet, after more than four years, I have not put needle to canvas! Maybe next winter!

I had been told that I could not use the ward payphone or have a shower because of the risk of infection from the mouthpiece of the phone and shower nozzle. One afternoon I was allowed to take a phone call from Helen. She was now convalescing at St Joseph's and she had wanted to let me know how well she was and how pleasant her stay was. That, of course, meant a hasty trip to Ward 7 to tell the staff of Helen's news.

On the morning of January 22nd I was drinking my mid-morning coffee when the sister came bustling in and said, "Don't have anything else to drink or eat. You're having a biopsy this afternoon!"

Once again I donned the obligatory white gown and off I was whisked to the angio suite. Part of this journey involved going in a lift – quite a tight squeeze for trolley, attendant nurse and porter. Coming out of the lift near the angio suite always worried me. There was a tight turn for a trolley from the lift, opposite a flight of stairs. I regularly had visions of the trolley with scantily-clad patient careering down those stairs.

This was the afternoon that Rob, a senior member of the school staff, was coming to see me. I had it all planned: I would be dressed and would meet him outside the ward so that he could let the staff at school know how well I was. Instead, when he came, there I was in bed, flat, unable even to sit up for three hours. However, it did mean that if the biopsy results were satisfactory, I would be home at the weekend.

Two days later I was told that the biopsy results were satisfactory. I immediately started to sort out the things which could go home with Alan when he came for his usual evening visit. I was surprised at how much I had accumulated during my stay in Room 2. I left all the cards on the walls until last, otherwise everywhere would look so bare – just as rooms do after the Christmas decorations are taken down.

I untaped my 'Teddy' – this was a pad of old pillowcases provided for those who have had open-heart surgery. The Teddy can be pressed to the chest to help the post-operative pain. As I never had any pain, my Teddy was used as an arm rest for my wooden-armed easy chair.

Mr Murday came and talked to Alan and me about the regime after the transplantation, including the forthcoming hospital visits.

On the morning of January 27th, four weeks after my transplant, I was all packed and eagerly waiting when Alan arrived at 10.30 to take me home.

Home!

No way was I cooking on that first day home, so we called at a local public house where I enjoyed a large Yorkshire pudding with onion gravy. It was a fine winter's day and at two o'clock, a reporter and a photographer appeared from the *Courier*. It was warm enough to have photographs taken with Alan in our garden. It was great to be able to breathe fresh air instead of the warm centrally-heated fug of the hospital. I had often sniffed fresher air when on my walks up and down stairs near the ward where a window was generally partially open, but it was not really fresh.

I made several phone calls to family and friends and revelled at being back home and once again sleeping in my own bed.

A number of visitors arrived during the following day with flowers, cards, and bulbs. I had my first walk outside. Fortunately we live near the 'White Lee recreation ground'. Gladys called for me and we walked around this area which is comparatively level for our 'Pennine Village'. So began my daily walk with Gladys, progressing a little further each day. Gladys became known as my minder and her support was invaluable.

On my second day at home, Alan took me by car up to school where I walked cautiously into the staff room during the daily morning meeting held for staff. David, the headmaster, was halfway through delivering a notice when he looked across, saw me and broke off, exclaiming in an amazed voice, "There's June Buckley."

I said, "I've come to say thank you for your support. I thought it was better to come personally than to write a letter."

I stayed talking to several staff for some time. One young teacher came up and said, very quietly, "I've been able to keep tabs on your progress through a friend of mine." Jon, the young teacher, lived in Leeds and knew someone who worked in the pharmacy department of the hospital. On the evening of my transplant she could not meet Jon as she was sorting out the drugs needed for the operation. She then gave regular progress reports to Jon who had relayed them to other members of staff.

After some time in school I walked home – on my own!

My GP called and asked a number of questions. He knew someone who had had a heart transplant now! He was followed by a reporter from the *Hebden Bridge Times* newspaper, which was quite a pleasant interlude as the reporter was an ex-pupil.

At times it was very quiet at home after the hustle, bustle and general noise in the hospital. I loved being at home.

January 30th was a very sad day. Julie, a nurse from Ward 7, phoned to tell me that Helen had died. She had been rushed back from St Joseph's but nothing could be done. Helen had fought so hard and was such a lovely person. We had made plans to meet and visit each other on her return home, but it was not to be. I am still in regular contact with her daughter Jackie.

I went shopping for the first time, with my minder of course. Everything seemed strange after three months away. I was frequently stopped in the village and asked how I was. Often the preamble began with, "Are you. . .?" or "Is it. . .?"

I made my first visit to the local library for months. I could now walk that far with ease. I felt that I could settle down and read a novel again. Flowers, cards and letters continued to arrive and I spent time daily arranging the blooms in my amateurish way.

I relished having leisurely baths in a warm bathroom. Oh, the joy of being able to rub myself dry instead of sitting on the edge of the bath with a towel wrapped round me, hoping I would get dry! I was also beginning to gain some weight and my skin was no longer hanging in 'elephant-like' folds from my arms and bottom.

I had been at home for a week when I was asked to take Hebden assembly. It felt strange standing up in front of almost three hundred staff and pupils again after a break of over two years. It was good to talk to the older pupils who I knew very well. The assembly itself was not memorable – I was sadly out of practice.

A break in my daily walks came about because of heavy snowfalls in the area. The hills took on a different appearance and looked extremely picturesque. Alan managed to take me by car to Leeds General Infirmary for my first of a number of weekly visits to Ward 23, where examinations including blood tests were done and steroid dosage adjusted accordingly. I still had the 'moonface' associated with taking steroids. Alan continued to refer to me as Hamster Features.

These weekly Wednesday morning trips to Leeds were stressful because of the traffic problems. Even though we left home before eight o'clock, traffic into Halifax had already built up. This became much worse as we approached the outskirts of Leeds. I was frequently late for my appointment. I was seen regularly by Mr Murday and on one occasion was given an invitation to his leaving party at a Leeds nightclub. This was a very noisy but pleasant evening spent in the company of two other transplantees and their wives. I danced too, just nine weeks after my transplant.

This ended our connection with Mr Murday, who was going to a London hospital where he could continue to perform transplant operations.

Alison and family were moving to live in America in the late spring, and as they were letting their house in England they came *en famille* to stay with us while their home was redecorated. On their arrival I was greeted by an excited Max who rushed in saying, "Grandma, Grandma, sit down and shut your eyes." I heard him staggering around and a box was dumped at my feet. There was a scrabbling noise and out popped two of the most delightful kittens imaginable – one tortoiseshell and the other black and white. I knew nothing about this surprise, though Alan did.

Apparently, when Alison had told Max that they were coming to Yorkshire, Max had said that he liked coming because of Grandma and the cat. He then said, "But Dennis has died."

"Yes," replied Alison, "She was a very old cat."

After a few minutes Max asked, "When we go to Yorkshire, can we take Grandma a present?"

"Of course." said Alison. "What do you want to take her?"

"A baby cat," was the reply.

Alison had then spoken to Alan and asked him what we would say to a kitten. Alan told her that we had planned to replace Dennis as we'd always had a cat. Alison made some enquiries and after a few days phoned again and asked, "How would you react to *two* kittens?" To which Alan replied, "Funnily enough, we had talked of having two kittens as company for each other."

"Well," said Alison, "I've heard of two kittens who have been fostered out prior to rehousing. Shall I go and see them?"

"Certainly," was Alan's answer.

That is how we acquired Topsy and Buttons. At first Max was very upset at the names, as he had already christened them Marian and Robin. However, Topsy and Buttons they are called. Alan named Topsy, the tortoise shell, because for years at his home there had been a tortoise shell cat called Topsy. It was left to me to name the black and white kitten. She had a white mask, probably where Robin came from (Batman and Robin). She had a tiny, pale, pink nose just like a button – hence her name. They have been a source of delight to us ever since. Thank you, Max and Alison.

My first visit to hospital after Mr Murday's departure was unfortunate. I sat with two other transplant patients for over two hours in a draughty area at the outpatients department waiting to be seen by a doctor we did not know and who didn't know us. I had developed a cold and had a temperature, so I was not happy. I came back home, but two days later as my temperature was still high it was back again to Leeds and Ward 7.

It was somewhat different this time. Ward 7 was mixed throughout. We had been asked for our opinions about this before my transplant and oddly enough it was the men who objected more than the women.

A biopsy showed that I had some rejection which I had vowed would *not* happen to me. A different drug regime started, including intravenous injections of steroids. Two more biopsy tests were undertaken in six days, then I was allowed home.

I felt really well again so life was back to normal – walking, shopping, and so on. I used to wake up in the mornings and think, I'm here. Whatever the weather, when anyone grumbled about it being a dreadful day, I would say and still do, "It's a wonderful day!" I got some peculiar looks from people.

My sixth biopsy, on April 2nd went well. On my return home I felt unwell. When I was not feeling any better the following morning, Alan phoned the local group practice surgery. When the doctor came, he said that I should be in hospital. I said, "Do I have to?" just like a child. He phoned the hospital and I overheard him say, "Resisting as usual."

Once again it was Ward 7. My throat was very sore and my mouth very painful. I found it extremely difficult and painful to eat. Tests showed that herpes had grown on top of ulcers in my mouth. A soft food diet was suggested. This consisted of mashed potatoes and mince, followed by shepherds pie, followed by mince and mashed potatoes, followed by. . . I finally asked if I could choose something from the trolley instead.

My temperature continued to go up and down erratically, until after being very high one night, a day of tests followed. This entailed travelling from one end of the large hospital to the other and back again for a lung function test, X-ray, Echo cardiogram, CT scan, and biopsy. In between all this, for three separate hours each day I was pinned down as I was attached to a drip stand.

During this stay, two of the 'gang' were also occupying beds on the ward – John because he was unwell and Ken for his first year's test (known as the MOT). It was then a year since I had first met Ken, when I was being assessed and he had just had a transplant.

After almost two and a half weeks I was on my way home again. I had sampled all four rooms which made up Ward 7, so I said that I would not be in again to stay. So far I have kept my word!

Hospital visits were now once a fortnight, and we were seen on Ward 7 by the doctors instead of in the Outpatients Department which we preferred. Generally there were three or four of the 'gang' present so we had an interesting time, joking and comparing notes. We were also provided with coffee – a bonus – even hospital coffee!

I had started going regularly again to the Calder Valley Club, working mostly in the kitchen, preparing vegetables, serving the lunches and washing up. On the odd occasion, though, Joan and I were called upon to cook the lunch for the members. We always enjoyed our day there.

Regularly on Wednesday mornings I went into school and worked in the special needs department, or rather went into normal classes and helped special needs pupils. I was asked to write the maths work for one boy who had his writing hand in a sling. I thought that this would be simple, as all I would have to do would be to write down his verbal answers. This was not so. His work involved co-ordinates which meant that there was a certain amount of measuring. One of the known side effects of the Cyclosporin drug is shakiness of the hands. I often wondered what that boy thought about me, having unsteady hands at nine-thirty in the morning.

The shakiness varied from day to day, until now it has virtually stopped. In the early days, coffee granules were regularly spilt when transferring the spoonful from coffee jug to mug, hence home-made soup was a disaster. The herbs and spices are kept in a cupboard near the hob, and I was in the habit of just reaching up and shaking a few of the chosen herbs into the bubbling pot without measuring them out. After a full carton of mixed herbs landed in the celery soup I started to use a teaspoon!

The growth of body hair was another side effect and I was not pleased to get a downy growth on my face. I made a visit to the helpful local chemist and a cream was recommended. It worked and still does. Those were the only two side effects which I had and have.

On Easter Sunday I decided to go to church. I went by car with Geoffrey and Gladys and enjoyed being able to sing the well-known hymns without being breathless. I walked happily to the altar rail for communion and then came a mini disaster. Trying to stand up again, I found that my leg muscles were still not strong enough. I very nearly knocked over the rail. Gladys came to my rescue and hauled me to my feet again.

This episode reminded me of another occurrence in hospital about two weeks after the transplant. I had gone to the refrigerator in the ward kitchen to fetch one of the high protein drinks which were on the bottom shelf. I bent down to choose a flavour I preferred but could not get up. After falling backwards onto my bottom I had to wait there until someone came.

Gardening was done daily, or when weather permitted. There was seed planting in the greenhouse and then the transplanting of seedlings, and finally the planting out. Our garden had been sadly neglected over the past year, so we were determined to have an extra colourful summer display. Alan and I decided to have a thank you day at home for all our friends and neighbours who had been so helpful and supportive to us both during the months of waiting and recovering. I planned to do the majority of the catering myself, and a date in early August was fixed.

It was now almost six months since the transplant and I decided to try and let my donor's family know how well I was and how thankful I was to be given a second chance of living.

I knew the donor had been a twenty-five-year-old woman who had been in a car accident in Hull. I phoned the Hull daily newspaper, asking the reporter if he thought that it would not upset the donor's relatives, could they be told how well I was and let them know that I was extremely grateful for their unselfish action which had enabled me to keep alive. I explained that in their position it would help me to grieve to know that some good had come out of such a tragic accident.

The reporter asked if he could have my name in case the family wished to contact me. I said no to this, and to the request for my phone number. Then he asked, "Where did your operation take place?" Without thinking, I answered, "Leeds General Infirmary."

The next day a *Halifax Courier* reporter phoned and said, "I hear you have been to Hull to find out about your donor." I denied this and explained why I had contacted the Hull paper and assumed that would be the end – not so. The following day the donor's details were published. I learnt that she had been a Dutch vet, working in Bridlington, going home to Holland for Christmas. The accident was on Christmas Eve, so she had been on a life support machine for four days. Her name was there also – I have deliberately not remembered it.

Two years later, while taking our cats for their yearly injections to our local veterinary surgery, the vet commented on how well I looked. I laughingly said, "Well, I got a good heart, it belonged to a vet!" Our vet had read all about the fatal accident in a veterinary magazine and said, "All the vets I know carry a donor card."

The health reporter from the *Yorkshire Evening Post* used to phone regularly to find out how I was, to get my views on the shortage of donors, and to chat about Norfolk, our home county. He enquired if I had had my longed-for balloon flight, to which I replied, "Not yet, but it is arranged."

That first meeting with this reporter, when I had just arrived at Room 2 from Intensive Care, had caught me by surprise. I was asked what I wanted to do when I was once again active. I had replied, "Have a hot air balloon flight, go to America and Canada to see my family, learn to tap dance, and live to the year 2000."

When this had appeared in the local newspaper, a friend of ours had said to his wife, "We must find out when June goes up in the balloon. I'd love to go up myself and I want to watch her flight!"

Unbeknown to Bill, Norah, his wife, had booked the balloon trip to coincide with Bill's sixty-fifth birthday and his retirement from work. I was going up with him – our birthdays were only one day apart.

The evening before *the* day was wet and windy, and the balloonist contacted Norah and said that the flight was cancelled.

Norah gave Bill the flight money on his birthday morning and told him what it was for. Alan and I had been invited to Bill's birthday lunch at a nearby restaurant and after that had gone back to their house for tea. We had just eaten and cut the balloon decorated cake when the phone rang. We heard Norah say, "Yes, we can. What time is it now?" With a huge smile she came into the room and said, "Now that the wind has dropped and the sky looks settled, the balloon flight is on. We've half an hour to get to the playing fields."

I've never seen a house empty so quickly as we piled into cars and made our way down the valley to the school playing fields in Mytholmroyd.

I had taken a change of suitable clothing with me, just in case, so I quickly changed into jeans and jumper covered with colourful balloons. Ian, Bill, and Norah's son had called in at his home and brought two leather flying helmets which we donned to have our photographs taken.

We watched the balloon being inflated, and so did the local cricket team who had finished their match. There were four of us in the basket, which was much larger than I expected. As well as Bill and myself, there was another woman who had been given a flight as a fortieth birthday present, and, of course, the balloonist himself. The take-off was so smooth that it was only when we were above the heads of the spectators that I realised we were up.

There was very little wind, so the movement in the balloon was only slight and we hardly seemed to be moving. We were in regular radio contact with the back-up team on the ground. They were told in which direction we were heading and which road to take by car.

It was so quiet and peaceful – the stillness only broken by the regular noise of the gas cylinders firing the flame. At one point we appeared to be going round in circles as the wind current altered. We drifted over a part of the valley with which I was unfamiliar, but we were given comments on landmarks and various features were pointed out to us by the balloonist. Tidy and untidy gardens, open air swimming pools, a dried-up reservoir, a golf course, and a large housing estate all passed beneath our floating canopy. Our line of following cars looked the size of Matchbox toys and we could see as far as the M62 motorway.

All too soon, the end of the hour's flight was near and our pilot was searching for somewhere to land. Most of the likely looking fields had farm animals in them, so these had to be avoided. Eventually we were told to brace ourselves for a landing which might be a bit bumpy. We were going to land in a hayfield. We had gathered quite a crowd of people who followed our descent on foot, bicycle and car.

The farmer who owned the hayfield came running out waving his arms and shouting, "Gerr off, Gerr off! Do you want a cup of tea?" His whole family came out to greet us and to share in our champagne.

They said that they had never seen so many people near their isolated farmhouse and they seemed to enjoy their unusual Sunday evening. "Better than watching telly," was a comment. We were given certificates which stated that we had made a 'maiden flight in *Bridesnightie.*' As soon as I asked why the balloon was so named I realised that I should have kept quiet!

After watching the balloon being deflated and packed away we all wended our way home. That was an experience, hopefully to be repeated some day, perhaps in a westerly rather than an easterly direction – all depending on the wind.

It was time for a six months' biopsy. I travelled to Leeds by train as we had found it less stressful than trying to get to the hospital in time for appointments by car. Alan fetched me home that same evening by car – traffic is so much lighter in the evenings although parking at the hospital is virtually impossible. We had our traffic warden contact who would move cones so that we could park near the Casualty entrance.

Two days after the biopsy the registrar phoned to say that there was some cellular infiltration showing up and that the slides from the biopsy were being sent to Mr Murday in London. The message received back said that there was nothing to worry about and medication was to continue as normal.

Meanwhile I had been preparing for our 'thank you' day. A large heart-shaped fruit cake was made and taken to be decorated by Hazel who specialised in icing cakes – not Hazel with the ankle problem, but Hazel with the knees! This Hazel had undergone two knee joint replacements twice!! The freezer was full of pies, pasties, and gateaux. Meat was cooked, carved and plated, wine and glasses were ordered, and the garage had been cleaned out and a bar arranged there.

It was a wonderful day and a beautiful, sunny, summer afternoon. One of the other Leeds transplantees and his wife came! Jo, the heart-and-lung wonder and her husband, nurses from Leeds, including my primary nurse, Martin, ex-patients I had come to know from both Halifax and Leeds hospitals, and a host of friends. I felt then that we had in some way managed to say thank you to so many people.

A few weeks after this, the annual 'Take Heart' sponsored walk took place in Rounday Park, Leeds. The 'Take Heart' club had been formed by ex-heart patients and their families as a support group. Fund raising for the cardiac wards in Leeds had become an important part of the club. One event which raises thousands of pounds is the sponsored walk. I decided to enter on September 1st, 1991. People could tackle a variety of distances from just over a mile to twelve miles. That day Alan and I walked six miles. One circuit was three miles, and after covering the same ground twice I decided that that was enough, not because I could not walk any more but because I do not enjoy going over the same ground again and again. I have always enjoyed walking, but I try not to come back by the same route as I set out on.

Calder High School sponsored me for the 'Take Heart' six miles and I handed over four hundred and fifty pounds to the club.

My next target was our visit to Canada and America to see both daughters. Alison was now living in the States, but she had seen me post transplant. Cheryl, though, living in Montreal, did not really know how I was. No matter how often I said over the phone that I was well, it was not the same as seeing me face to face. I had been told by the doctors that I could travel, but I was advised not to go in the heat of the summer, which was why we were travelling at the end of September. I was armed with a letter from the consultant which stated that I was fit to travel. Alison had contacted the hospital in Indianapolis enquiring if they could cope with me in an emergency. We were informed that a hospital in Montreal was apparently one of the finest for cardiac treatment in the world.

The cats were left in the capable hands of Geoffrey so that they could stay in their familiar surroundings, and off we went. Our flight was from Manchester to Toronto, where we were to be met by ex-teaching colleagues from way back who had emigrated to Canada the year we moved from Southend on Sea to Yorkshire. We were delayed at the airport though, as for some reason Alan and I were singled out by Customs officers for questioning.

Rather stupidly, Alan had told the huge, bored-looking customs officer that we were both carrying a quantity of drugs. The man immediately straightened up and stared at us.

"Yes," said Alan. "Cyclosporin for one. My wife should not be kept standing around."

"Oh," commented the official, "Transplant, I suppose. Go that way." He indicated another exit.

Feeling very relieved, we walked through to the main concourse and saw our friends searching for us, assuming we would be coming through the proper exit. Being well over six feet tall, Dick was easy to spot.

Whoever we told about Alan's facetious comments to the customs officer came up with the same remark, "You should never have said that. No one messes with Customs officers. They haven't a sense of humour."

We spent an enjoyable few days some miles out from Toronto, marvelling at Dick's house which he had built himself, and sampling the facilities of Port Hope before returning to nearby Toronto for a brief stay with Ann. Ann and I had started primary school together at the age of four. I had not seen her for years, so we sat and talked and reminisced for hours. We were taken to Niagara Falls, a truly magnificent sight.

Flying on to Montreal, we spent our time with Cheryl and our two grandsons.

We met her friends and work colleagues who until then had just been names to us. The autumn was beginning and the colours of the trees were as brilliant as I had imagined and expected.

We even went to a parents' evening at Matthew's secondary school – a coals-from-Newcastle affair for us. It was a similar experience, which we knew so well, except that half of the lessons were spoken in French. Teachers were inclined to speak in French to us until we spoke in English.

Cheryl lives in an apartment, and looking out of a window to another three-storey apartment block I was amazed to see a squirrel climb up a sheer brick wall, stopping off at various window sills to see if there was anything edible for him before coming down to ground level again. Squirrels are prolific in that part of Montreal. We thought them delightful, but Cheryl dismissed them as vermin.

From Montreal we flew to Indianapolis where Alison and her family were now living with their three cats and large pointer dog. Everything here was on a big scale and completely geared to the motor car with drive-in banks, cinemas, McDonalds, and so on. No one walked if they could go by car. When Alan and I went for a walk along the avenue where they lived, we never met anyone else walking. It seemed strange to us.

On our return to England we had to change planes at Atlanta. Tony, our son-in-law, said to me, "There's no way you are going to walk from the domestic terminal to Atlanta's continental terminal, so I'll arrange for you to be met when you land."

"I'll be all right," I replied. "I'm fine!" I had recently walked six miles. I thought, 'what's he *fussing* about!'

"I fly into Atlanta regularly," said Tony, "and I know what it is like!"

I decided to do as the doctor said!

During the short flight from Indianapolis to Atlanta, a stewardess came up to me and said, "You are Mrs Buckley and I believe you need a wheelchair when we land, so please wait until all the passengers have disembarked."

"I don't need a wheelchair," I protested. "I can walk all right but maybe not a long distance."

"Oh," she said, "Would a buggy do, then? If so, I'll phone ahead and let the airport know."

Sure enough, a chirpy attendant and an electric buggy which had a continuously tinkling bell was waiting for us. We were taken with our luggage quite a distance to a lift at the bottom of which we were met by a minibus and an equally cheerful man who took us right across runways to the other terminal. I was so pleased that we had not had to find our own way.

Arriving home, we found that our cats had been so well looked after by Geoffrey that they didn't really make a fuss of us, much to my disappointment. They both looked fat and contented. It had been arranged that we would have our evening meal on our return at Geoffrey and Gladys' house. There was a note from Geoffrey saying that the meal was off because Gladys was ill. Bell's Palsy had been diagnosed, so we went to see her before opening all the junk mail which had accumulated in our absence or attending to our luggage.

Gladys did not look at all well and she had been such a tower of strength to us both, doing shopping, ironing, visiting me regularly in hospital, walking with me daily and providing meals for Alan. Subsequently the prognosis was a mild stroke. Gladys has recovered remarkably well and is back to her jovial, jolly self.

Instead of one of Gladys' lovely meals I had to delve into the freezer for food. By evening the cats had forgiven us for deserting them. Both of them spent the night on our bed, fussing around us for ages.

It was my turn to do shopping for Gladys and to have her and Geoffrey over for a meal or two. Quite often, when I was in the village or even at nearby Hebden Bridge, I would be asked, "Where's your minder?" This was often followed by "How's Gladys?" Gladys had lived and worked locally all her life, so she was well known.

I still had my main housework done for me. I was so used to having my cleaning done that I didn't fancy doing it again. Of course, prior to my transplant I was incapable of wielding a vacuum cleaner, and help was a necessity; now it is a luxury which I still thoroughly enjoy.

Weekly visits to the Calder Valley Club and the school were continued. Life was wonderful! Hospital visits were now once a month. My first-year tests were approaching, but before that I went for breast screening.

When asked by the nurse if I had any problems, I replied, "yes."

"What?" was the interested question.

"Finding them," I replied. "I've never been well blessed in that department."

"Don't worry, we'll find them," was the answer.

When I went into the little room for the X-ray, I was told by the doctor, "I'd rather have you than the previous lady, as I couldn't get all her breast on the plate." She then said, "I know what that scar is," pointing to the one down the middle of my chest, "but what is the one going across?" She indicated the pacemaker scar. At least she had read my notes beforehand, unlike the nurse when I had gone for a cervical smear before the transplant operation.

Alan and I made an extra journey to Leeds General Infirmary one afternoon, when a special trolley was handed over to the cardiac wards, thanks to the proceeds from the 'Take Heart' sponsored walk. As well as the money raised by the pupils at my old school, the head of boys' physical education had run the Calderdale Way, aided by some of the staff, and had collected another hundred pounds, so that also went to the 'Take Heart Club'.

On the morning of December 16th I left home at the unearthly hour of half past six so that I could be in hospital at Leeds for my first year tests that morning. When I had asked what time I needed to be there, the nurse had replied, "Seven-thirty."

"You're joking," I said.

But she wasn't. I had been so worried about not hearing the alarm clock or because it might not ring that I kept waking up, and finally I got up before five o'clock. Instructions were: nothing to eat or drink after midnight, so I could not even have a cup of coffee. I cleaned my teeth twice so that my mouth did not feel so dry. It felt very strange walking to the station at that early hour. A milk float and a large lorry were all the traffic I saw.

My MOT, which involved an angiogram and another biopsy, went well. I saw quite a·few people I knew, although there were some strange faces amongst the nursing staff. After one night's stay on Ward 7, I was home again, looking forward to Christmas and my first anniversary. I had been in the habit of counting the months that first year.

Now on December 28th or 29th we do something to celebrate, but that first December we had eight friends to spend the evening with us. I think an enjoyable evening was had by all. It seemed a fitting end to my first year after. . .

1992 started well. How did I ever find time to work full time? I was asked to do some English coaching for a few pupils and also for an Indian lady. She had been to America to visit a brother who told her that her spoken English was poor. Very tentatively, she asked if I could help her and I agreed and I soon found out that her English, particularly grammar, was excellent. I think the only way I helped her was to give her confidence when speaking. I certainly learned a great deal about her life in India.

An exercise-to-music class started in the village for people of various ages, abilities and disabilities. I decided to join, having first obtained permission from the medics. We were, and still are, a motley collection of people, but we do enjoy our Tuesday morning sessions.

I think it's truly amazing how some people cope. Because of this one session, I thought I could really do with a second weekly dose of exercise so I started to attend a women's keep fit class each Thursday evening. This was also held locally. I want to try tap dancing, but so far I haven't found a class suitably near my home.

The Transplant Games in 1992 were being held at Exeter and I particularly wanted to go, as our elder daughter had been a student in Exeter, a city we all liked. Leeds General did not have a team and I could not get seconded to another hospital team in time, so I had to miss out.

I continued to walk nearly every day, often along the canal bank to Hebden Bridge. There are some lovely walks in our area; nearly all can be circular. Woods and hills, moors and farmland all add to the variety. There are numerous rivers, streams and reservoirs to complement the land.

On Sunday in mid-February, Alan and I joined the Take Heart Walking Club who were walking the canal bank from Todmorden to Hebden Bridge, where a pub lunch had been booked. It was a lovely brisk winter's day. After lunch, the walkers continued walking by the canal to Mythonroyd and came to our house for further refreshments before catching a train back to Leeds. Forty pairs of boots and shoes lined up outside the front door caused a number of comments. It was an enjoyable day. The only problem had been from the number of cyclists riding along the bank, many of whom gave no warning of their approach.

Opening a letter one morning, I was startled to find that I was being asked to open Mythonroyd Gala in the summer. I had worked in the catering department of this annual event for a number of years but I had no idea what the opener did. When I was in the surgery collecting my monthly pill prescription, I saw my GP and asked if I could speak to him privately. He and his wife had opened the gala one year. He just roared with laughter and said, "Enjoy the day and wear comfortable shoes."

I must admit that I *did* enjoy my day and I did wear flat, comfortable shoes, but I prefer my usual position on the outside catering stall. However, that year I had time to speak to people, to wander from stall to stall, be amazed at the number of people involved or attending the event and the variety of stalls and entertainment. A reporter I knew from the *Courier* asked me what I thought of the event and he said that he had to attend most such occasions in Calderdale, and the Mythonroyd Gala was by far the best. It raises vast sums of money for the benefit of local societies.

Jo had her fortieth birthday in May and she had a party to celebrate reaching this milestone, one she thought she would never see. Many of the people at this momentous event were patients from Papworth, who had undergone, or were waiting for heart or lung operations.

Monthly visits to the hospital continued, but after one journey by car which took us over two and half hours to cover the twenty-two and a half miles, I decided that further visits would be by train. It also meant that Alan did not need to take time off work. The last late visit had meant that the doctor had been to the ward and gone, likewise the 'vampire' trolley and attendant and the ECG equipment. I had to chase all over the hospital, or so it seemed, to have the necessary tests.

I mentioned the train idea to Joan, who immediately said, "I'll come with you. After the hospital business we can shop in Leeds and have some lunch there." Trust British Rail? Never! The train was over half an hour late at Mytholmroyd and was further delayed at subsequent stations. Seeing a policeman on the concourse of Leeds station, Joan asked him the quickest way to the infirmary, to which he replied, straight-faced, "Walk under a bus," before proceeding to give proper instructions. On our return to the station some hours later the same policeman was still there. I walked up to him. "We found our way," I told him, "*without* the bus."

In mid-June Alison and family came from the States for a holiday. It was lovely to see them again. My sixtieth birthday arrived and what a day that was. I was not allowed to open any cards until lunchtime and presents were quickly whizzed away. I was busy opening cards when Alison bustled into the room with, "Hurry up, we're going out!"

"Where?"

"Never mind, just come and get into the car."

We set off on what was for me a mystery trip. We reached and passed Skipton and I wondered if another balloon trip was the surprise. We left the balloon centre behind and arrived at Giggleswick. Apart from the public school and Russell Harty, I knew nothing about Giggleswick. Then I saw a sign which read:

YORKSHIRE DALES, FALCONRY AND CONSERVATION CENTRE. What a treat! We looked at various birds of prey, watched a free-flying demonstration before going into the tea-room. My favourite owl of all is the Barn Owl, and usually Barney is in the tea-room to entertain but he wasn't there that day. The catering staff had made a chocolate cake instead, iced and decorated as an owl.

On our return home, Chris and his family arrived and I was finally allowed to open my presents. From the whole family I had a large box which contained sixty numbered parcels. Max handed me the numbered presents, hardly giving me time to open it before handing the next one to me. It was all bewildering. We then went to an Italian restaurant for a family meal. Just as we had finished, a waitress appeared carrying a silver salver on which sat a foil swan decorated with red carnations. There was a small box nestling between the swan's wings.

"What's that?" I asked Alan.

"Probably After Eight mints, but open it and see for yourself." The waitress was still hovering by my side as I undid the wrapped box. It didn't contain chocolates but a ruby and diamond eternity ring. Alan's present. What a surprise!

On returning home once again, the day was completed when I spoke to Cheryl in Montreal. I'll never forget my sixtieth birthday.

More sad news came when John died. He was one of the most cheerful and full-of-fun characters I've ever met. He had had a heart transplant a few months before me. I knew his joking personality hid a frightened and worried man, but he always managed to make me laugh. He had been to our home a few times and we frequently met in Leeds. The last time I had seen him was while he was a patient on Ward 7 and he was moved temporarily out of his bed into a wheelchair while three of us were examined. He was still joking, making comments about us being in his bed, and chatting up the nurses. John had been very depressed because of his inability to find employment. He had had a responsible job with a large transport firm prior to being ill, but whatever work he had applied for he rarely got an interview. On one occasion John had been interviewed and was recalled for a second interview. When he was asked why he'd been unemployed for two years, John said that he'd been redecorating his home.

"For two years?" came the query.

"If I said I'd had time off ill, would that prejudice my chances?" asked John.

"What was wrong?" asked the interviewer.

"A bypass operation," and then, looking the man behind the desk straight in the eyes, he added, "and a heart transplant."

John said that a certain look came into the man's eyes, so John stood up, saying, "Thank you for the coffee," and walked out. He had applied for over thirty jobs.

The rest of us all met at his funeral, plus some of the nursing staff and 'hairy' Malcolm, who was back teaching after his successful bypass.

Ken had met similar prejudice when seeking employment and had also applied and been rejected many times. As a joiner he managed to get some work for a while, purely by chance. Ken had been walking past a disused cinema which was being converted into something else, when he heard banging. Going in, he asked the foreman if he needed a joiner and when the answer was yes, Ken said that he would need one day off every month for a hospital check-up as he had had a heart transplant. The foreman asked if it would prevent Ken from working normally: if not, he could start straightaway.

For some time, Gladys had handed on to me the *Woman's Weekly* magazine which in turn had been passed on to her. I used to flick through them generally, reading the letters' page, perusing recipes and knitting patterns and any articles which appealed to me. Glancing through one of these magazines, I was attracted by the word 'trampolining' and looked a bit closer at the article. The name Glenda appeared but with a surname I did not recognise. When I worked in Southend on Sea, my most successful trampoline pupil was a girl called Glenda. There was a photograph of Glenda with a group standing by a trampoline in the magazine.

It was a 'True to Life' story relating how Glenda, a trampoline coach, had overtwisted when trampolining and had broken her neck. After months of hospital treatment she was almost back to normal, but could no longer bounce on the trampoline. I had not seen Glenda since she was a fifteen-year-old schoolgirl. Now she was married with four children, some of whom were British trampoline champions in their age groups. I decided to write to her via Southend Education Authority as the magazine stated she was a teacher in the town. I was dismayed when the letter was returned as 'unknown'! Writing a covering letter to the magazine, I enclosed my original missive asking the editor to forward it to Glenda.

A few days later I received a reply from Glenda and we have been in regular contact since. Glenda's eldest son is a student at Manchester, so when she comes north to visit him we often get a visit.

Gladys belongs to the Calder Valley Flower Club and was asked to do an arrangement in a local house for Cancer Charity. I started thinking that if money could be raised that way, then maybe I could have our house decorated for the Heart Fund. I had already decided to try and raise some money for the *Yorkshire Evening Post*'s 'Have a Heart' appeal. Having talked over the idea with Alan and Gladys, I then tentatively approached a local NAFAS (National Association of Flower Arrangers Society) judge, Miss Brenda Gande, and was delighted when Brenda was so enthusiastic. First of all, we decided on a name so that a bank account could be opened. 'Hearts and Flowers' seemed an appropriate title. The dates set were August 6th to 8th 1993, almost a year hence. We then mulled over ideas until the start of 1993.

Not being a flower arranger myself, I was somewhat disconcerted when I was asked to do an arrangement at the flower festival in St Michael's Church, our local church. I hasten to explain that I was only asked because someone was ill. The theme throughout was Saints, and I was fortunate to be asked to portray St Francis. I have always liked Paul Gallico's book, *The Small Miracle*, where a small boy got papal consent to take his sick donkey into the crypt at Assisi. A special entrance had to be made to enable Pepino to get Violetta into the crypt. Part of the wall collapsed and St Francis' treasure box was revealed nestling in a niche. When the box was opened, it contained. . . a piece of hempen cord, knotted as though, perhaps, once it had been worn about the waist. Caught in the knot, as fresh as if it had grown but yesterday, was a single sprig of wheat. Dried and preserved, there also lay the stem and starry flower of a mountain primrose, and next to it one downy feather from a tiny meadow bird!

We had a suitable wooden box in which an approximation of the above articles was placed, and Alan wrote out the treasure description in his attractive italic handwriting. My actual floral arrangement was not very successful, as I could not get the gladioli to stay where I wanted them; however, the toy animals and birds I used proved popular.

With the prospect of having, hopefully, hundreds of people around our home we thought it was time we finally got the house in good repair. The priority was the roof. It had really needed re-roofing when we had moved in eleven years before. As it was a listed building we had to obtain the necessary permission from the Council. Some of the roof timbers needed replacing, but fortunately not too many of the stone slates. The house was built in 1727.

We had previously acquired the land at the rear of our house. This was bulldozed so that materials needed for the roof could be brought in that way. I watched with amazement as a large JCB was manoeuvred, flattening trees, large shrubs, greenhouses and walls, as though by a giant's hand. This was the start of many months of having workmen both outside and inside the house. I became a permanent tea and coffee maker.

Once the re-roofing was completed, the decorating could commence, since apart from the kitchen and downstairs cloakroom we had done no decorating at all. Nothing had needed doing when we moved in; I could not cope then with the upheaval involved, but now I was here to stay and work could commence. The bathroom was the first to receive the treatment, followed by hall, landing, and staircase, three bedrooms, the sitting-room, and exterior. Needless to say, we haven't had any more decorating done since those hectic months. There are still three rooms to go, plus the cellar and garage!

Life continued as normal amidst all the upheaval. I had started reading the local weekly newspaper to an elderly lady who was registered blind. The afternoons were and still are delightful. Edith is so amusing and has so many memories of days gone by and about people and events that are mentioned in the press.

There was nothing usual about the late evening of November 5th. We had kept both cats indoors until we assumed that the fireworks were over. I had gone to bed and was awakened by Alan shaking me and saying that something had happened to Buttons. Alan had heard

Buttons crying at the back door, and on opening it she had crept in dragging her tail.

I stumbled downstairs, and there was Buttons huddled against the radiator. Her tail looked like a piece of wet red string with a poodle's pom-pom at the end. We thought at first that it was the result of a firework, but there was no smell or singed fur. Trying to contact a vet at eleven o'clock on a Saturday night was no easy task. Our own vet was not answering our phone call – all we heard was the dreaded answerphone. We started on the Yellow Pages, going down the list of veterinary surgeons until one call was answered by a person in a car. This Halifax-based vet arranged to meet us at the surgery, so bundling up Buttons in a blanket, we set off.

Buttons was to lose her tail, the tail she loved to try and catch. We were told that she had been run over by a car – this was indicated by the fact that the fur which was stripped was the width of a car tyre and her front claws were worn down where she had tried to grip the road and escape.

We returned home somewhat subdued with instructions to telephone mid-afternoon on Monday to find out how Buttons was.

The hands of the clock did not seem to move on Monday afternoon, and at two o' clock I could wait no longer. I will never forget the reply to my query about Button's welfare. The receptionist said, "Oh, Buttons, she's fine but she does want to come home." Alan was working and could not get home until five o'clock at the earliest, so I phoned Joan with the news. She immediately said, "I'll come with you to collect Buttons, if you like." *If I liked*!

We brought home a very relieved and subdued cat with a stapled stump of a tail. For a few days she sat down somewhat tentatively.

The lack of a tail does not appear to worry Buttons now. She tends to wag her stump, reminiscent of a boxer or other dog with a docked tail. She no longer, as far as we can tell, goes across the road as she has a healthy respect for motorised vehicles.

December arrived and the time for my second year MOT. Once again, it was the early-morning trek to Leeds. Everything went smoothly until I got back to the ward. I stretched backwards over my prone position to reach my watch. The ward clock was not working and I didn't want to be flat any longer than necessary.

Whether it was because of the stretching or not – I assume it was – I started to bleed profusely from the femoral artery, which had been cut. I called a nurse and she pressed very heavily on my thigh for over half an hour. We were both somewhat bloody, as was the bed. The result of the excess bleeding was that I had to stay in hospital overnight. I was told that I could expect a little bruise.

The 'little' bruise took a few days to show itself in its true colours and it stretched from my groin to below the knee. The marks of the nurse's fingers were clearly visible, and my leg turned the colour of crushed blackberries. It was also somewhat uncomfortable. However, it did not prevent me enjoying Christmas and my second year party.

1993 was dominated by two events for me: the Transplant Games and the Flower Festival.

At the start of the year we made lists of businesses and societies who could be approached to give a donation in money or kind. A suitable letter was produced, thanks to one of Brenda's workmates. It was decided to ask members of flower clubs throughout East Lancashire and West Yorkshire to do an arrangement. This, of course, involved a vast amount of work for Brenda and a small committee, who had to decide where arrangements could be placed throughout the house. We ended up with flowers in every room, and my house plants filled the bath.

The local community, in particular, was extremely supportive and generous with donations and gifts for raffles and tombolas. Publicity was readily given by the press, although some was incorrect. It was stated that I planned to raise twenty thousand pounds, the cost of the operation, which was *never* my aim. I had only thought of a thousand pounds or so, as a thank-you gesture. Money is needed for so many good causes nowadays.

The Hearts and Flowers bank balance grew steadily, and every post brought money or something. Large stores and companies were on the whole not supportive, but they have regular charity commitments and Hearts and Flowers was not a registered charity.

We had regular meetings about the flower festival, and by mid-February, most of the letters had been sent and personal invitations had been given out to guests for the Friday preview evening, when wine and refreshments would be served. Joan Laprell, who writes in the *Lancashire and Yorkshire Ridings* magazine, agreed to open the event. She also lives locally and years before I had taught English to her younger son.

There was certainly plenty to keep me occupied; so many people helped that it would be impossible to mention them all by name.

I keep up my regular commitments: listening to reading at the local primary school, two lessons of Keep Fit and Aerobics, attending the Church Guild meetings and Calderdale newly-formed heart care meeting, reading to Edith, providing refreshments for the workmen, walking with Jo, and gardening, both at home and for Alan's and Geoff's gardening business. Like so many retired people, I could truly say, "I don't know how I found time to work."

A viewing afternoon and evening brought me face to face with the arrangers for the first time. I held a coffee morning in the village which raised well over a hundred pounds. The same morning that I had a letter from the area Freemasons saying that they would donate five hundred pounds to Heart and Flowers, I was stopped in the village by an elderly disabled lady who gave me five pounds. Wonderful gestures!

All the publicity stated that the Hearts and Flowers proceeds would go to the *Yorkshire Evening Post*'s 'Have a Heart' appeal. Three weeks before the actual festival, an early morning phone call came from the assistant editor of the *Yorkshire Evening Post* stating that the fund was closing and all money already raised were to be frozen. This decision had come about because of the national shortage of donors. In future, organs were to go only to designated transplant centres.

I felt both annoyed and upset. Was I going to get money under false pretences? I certainly did not want money I had raised to be frozen. Phone calls to the consultant cardiologist and the 'Take Heart' secretary in Leeds cooled me down and reassured me. Fortunately, the bank account was in the name of 'Hearts and Flowers', so money could go to the cardiac wards at Leeds General Infirmary. What a relief!

The week of the Flower Festival arrived – chaos! The decorators had not quite finished. Alan had designed a new front path to replace the cracked and broken concrete monstrosity. This incorporated a flower with a heart-shaped flag either side – very symbolic. The flower has since become Alan's trademark. Will he rival the mouse man, the Wharfedale wood carver?

Three days' raffles and tombolas were sorted, ticketed, and placed ready in boxes. Plants and ornaments were put out of the way, furniture was moved to accommodate floral arrangements, and everywhere was tidied. My wonderful cleaning lady thoroughly cleaned the house, and the garden was tidied and inspected for weeds. The garage had a mighty spring clean, resulting in a massive bonfire. Hopefully, we were ready.

Some of the arrangers had opted to come on Thursday evening to set up their displays, with the main group arriving on Friday morning. For a time there were people everywhere with boxes of greenery and flowers, but by mid-afternoon the house was quiet, sweet smelling and looking beautiful. Alan was frantically doing last minute work in the garden.

Alison and Rhiannon came late afternoon and four-year-old Rhiannon was the star of the show. Clad in a rose-sprigged party dress with a matching hat, she decided to station herself at the gate, on which the first of fifty floral decorations was placed, and usher in people. The first to arrive was Lady Thompson, the wife of our local MP. Sir Donald was on parliamentary business in Scotland. In his letter he had said that thanks to Leeds General Infirmary, he was *unable* to be present as he himself had recently recovered from a heart bypass operation at Leeds.

As Rhiannon brought her in, Lady Thompson apologised for being early and then said, smiling, "This little girl tells me that her teacher is called Mrs Thompson, so we have the same name."

I said, "But this is *Lady* Thompson, not *Mrs* Thompson." Rhiannon puzzled over this and obviously did not understand the difference between the two titles.

The house seemed all of a sudden full of people and chatter. Joan Laprell declared the festival open. There were so many people that I hardly spoke to anyone properly. I certainly did not eat much of the delightful bite-sized savouries and cakes. I should have secreted a plateful away before the proceedings began.

The raffle was drawn, the tombola table was cleared, and the evening was over. Money was counted, bagged, and taken to the bank's night safe. Bed beckoned.

I could not sleep, and finally at three o'clock I gave up the attempt and got up. The day's raffle was set up, sandwiches were taken from the freezer to defrost so that helpers would have something to eat. Refreshments today and Sunday were tea, coffee and biscuits. Marjory came to spray water over the arrangements, and Gladys to dust. Once again, we were ready.

There was a steady flow of visitors all day and the visitors' book contained many names and addresses.

Sunday was a much quieter day, but as far as I could tell everything went smoothly. The flowers were auctioned off at the end of the day – not a satisfactory affair as so many people had left. We had not thought that part out properly.

The weather had been reasonable without being brilliant. It had been quite windy, and unfortunately one outdoor arrangement was partially demolished. The plant stall was not over popular, neither were the china mugs depicting the Hearts and Flowers logo. Guessing the names of a brown bear (Boris), a clown (Buttons), and a gardener doll (Greenroyd), caused some hilarity. A beautiful, decorated, fruit cake had its weight accurately estimated. One bedroom was given over to a display of marquetry and landscape and floral pictures and cards. Jo's husband, Phil, is a keen photographer and his work attracted numerous customers. I also have a permanent record of the event, thanks to Phil. The smell of lavender bags and pot-pourri permeated the house for some days.

Altogether, over six hundred people came through the house that weekend, mainly women. Many friends provided invaluable help – involving visitors, supervising rooms, serving refreshments, washing up, selling raffle tickets and tombola tickets, making signs and labels, designing posters and programmes, and so on. I certainly could not have managed without those helping hands. Thank you all.

Suddenly it was all over. I had the task of contacting raffle prize winners who had not been present at the draw. On Thursday morning Gladys and Marjory arrived to vacuum and dust. What friends to have!

At the count-up I had far exceeded my original aim of a thousand pounds or so. The Hearts and Flowers bank account held well over three thousand pounds.

As previously mentioned, the other big event for me in 1993 was my visit to Newcastle and Gateshead for the 16th British Transplant Games. Killingbeck Hospital, also in Leeds, allowed me to join their team as a guest. On a fine morning in July two weeks before the Flower Festival Alan and I set out for our hotel in Newcastle, and after settling in made our way to the stadium in Gateshead, as I had entered for the mini-marathon in the veterans' class. Pounding the streets of Gateshead was not easy, but we were cheered on by marshals and spectators. It certainly seemed a long, hard three miles. A silver medal was my reward. There were only two competitors in the veterans' class! My number for the entire games was 513, so it was as well that I am not superstitious.

When I mentioned what I had done to an ex-teaching colleague, Rob, on my return, he asked, "Would you have done that if you hadn't had a transplant?"

I replied, "Running around the streets of Gateshead at my age? Don't be daft!"

The hospitality of the people of the north-east and the organisation was exceptional. We had a visit to Beamish Open Air Museum and another to a nature reserve. There was transport to take us from hotel to event or outing and back again, throughout our four-day stay.

Sunday was the main athletics day with competitors ages ranging from under three to over seventy. This is one meeting when the taking part, or the ability to take part, is the most important criterion, *not* the winning, although of course it is always satisfying to win. The morning of the two-mile walk saw the largest number of entries ranging from serious, competitive walkers to afternoon strollers. There was plenty of cheerful banter as we made our way out of the stadium along the designated route. The stadium was filling up with other competitors, relatives, transplant co-ordinators, medics, and friends. Everyone was cheerful as they re-entered the stadium. There was a bronze medal for me this time, and there were many in the veterans' class for this event.

We had managed to find seats in the stand near to the finish of the track races so we had a very good view. Joan and Kevin, her husband, had come for the weekend in the area and had joined us for the day.

There are three things which stand out particularly in my memory of that day. All the hospital teams participating paraded around the track in alphabetical order and lined up under their name in the centre of the stadium, just like at the Olympic and similar games. As we stood there I looked round and thought: There are over seven hundred of us here, so seven hundred people have died so that we can be here, *but if they had not died we would not be here.* It was a very sobering thought.

Secondly, watching a senior men's race, it was a joy to watch such a good athlete running and winning. But as soon as he had finished he ran almost halfway across the track to urge on another team competitor. We could hear him calling, "You can do it, you can do it," to the man who was jogging round.

Thirdly, there were the little children. One particular race is known as the Toddler's Dash. Generally, a parent is at the start of the thirty metre line, with the other parent or a nurse at the finishing line urging on their child. Perhaps a child runs with the parent or is even carried. Many spectators were in tears as they realised what those little children had had to endure already in their short lives.

After a gala dinner that evening, we were taken back to our hotels for our last night in Newcastle, returning home the following morning after a memorable four days. I was already looking forward to the 1994 games which were to be held in Portsmouth.

Visits to Leeds General Hospital were now only every three months, and I still went to the Royal Halifax Infirmary every six months. When I asked if I still needed to attend Halifax, the consultant said yes, so that my details would be readily available if needed. He then said, "We'll call it a social visit!"

When my name was called the very next time I was at the chest clinic, the staff nurse said, "In there, Mrs Buckley," indicating a small consulting room I knew well.

"What for?" I asked.

"So that the doctor can examine you, of course," she replied.

"But—" That was as far as I managed, as the nurse had hurried away.

I duly undressed to the waist and sat on the bed, waiting. The consultant bustled in with a cheery "Good morning, and how are you? Do you mind if two students come in as well?"

"No, not at all," I replied. "I'm fine, but I have a bone to pick with you."

"Oh, what's that?"

"At my age, when I go for a social visit," I said, looking him straight in the face, "I don't *strip.*"

Our cats are a continual source of pleasure, but one night Topsy did not come in, no matter how often she was called. The next morning we saw her stretched out on the path near the kitchen window. She could not get up and cried loudly when I picked her up and carried her indoors. After two days, during which she appeared to be no better, we took her to the vet. We left her for X-rays, and when we collected her later that day we were told that she had broken her pelvis in two places. Topsy, whom we knew crossed the road regularly, had also been hit by a car. Like Buttons, she had been very lucky – hopefully it will continue.

I had decided to have my third year MOT after Christmas. I didn't fancy having a large bruise and a tender leg at a busy time of year again. 1993 ended with Christmas being spent with Alison and family. Early in 1994, the MOT took place, fortunately with very little bruising this time. For the first time, the doctors and nurses did not wear masks and hats, as tests had shown them to be unnecessary for angiography and the like. It was a change to see their faces, instead of eyes only. They certainly looked more human, especially when they grimaced.

The day after that MOT, I met two primary schoolgirls for a press photograph. They were two non-stop chatterers and gigglers who had decided to hold a sponsored silence and raise some money. Both the photographer and myself wondered how on earth they had managed to stay silent for their designated time of one hour.

When Joan Laprell had opened the flower festival, she had asked if she could write an article about me for the *Lancashire and Yorkshire Ridings* magazine entitled, 'Women who achieve'. I had agreed and then forgotten all about it. One morning in February Joan came and the interview duly took place, with the article appearing in later editions of the magazines. The 'achiever' who came after me was Helen Sharman, the astronaut. She really is an achiever, in my opinion.

Several times since my article appeared I have been greeted by, "When I was in the dentist's waiting room [or doctor's waiting room, the hairdresser's, or the hotel lounge], I opened a magazine and there you were."

On my May visit to hospital in Leeds, I gave a cheque for three thousand, six hundred pounds to the two sisters on the cardiac wards so that they could buy something that was needed. I had reasoned that I had not wanted money raised going to the 'frozen' *Yorkshire Evening Post*'s appeal, but I was doing the same thing, so it was time to let the hospital have what money I had so far raised. It was several months before I learned what had been chosen with the money – bedside furniture and Aero Thermo Servo Humidifier Heaters and probe sensors.

I volunteered to read at a crèche one afternoon a week, which was an entirely different experience for me. The only times I had read to such young children was when our three children were young, or to our grandchildren. However, just as ever, some stories were wanted again and again and others were not liked at all.

One little girl, instead of playing with the toys and equipment provided, wanted me to read all the time. I looked forward to those afternoons, but unfortunately the group no longer functions.

Jo came regularly for our monthly walks. Try as we might to follow a map, we usually went wrong, but so far we have always got safely back. We generally walked between six and eight miles, talking constantly and eating a picnic lunch somewhere *en route*.

One morning we, or rather Jo and her husband, had carefully planned our route, so we set off confidently. As usual, we took a wrong turning somewhere on the open moor, landing up at the wrong reservoir. We walked some way around this reservoir before meeting a solitary man. We all said, "Good afternoon," and carried on walking. Suddenly the man called out "June," and turning round I recognised Geoff. He used to live in the valley and some years ago had moved to Cornwall. He had returned for a short holiday. Meeting him by an isolated moorland reservoir was truly amazing.

Jo asked me if I would take part in the Wharfedale Heart Research walk on Ilkley Moor. I agreed. We started off in brilliant sunshine, which was a problem as it was difficult seeing the rocks and boulders with the sun gleaming on my glasses. We ended up in 'stair rod' rain. Thirteen miles of moorland were covered that day. Walking through tussocky heather is not particularly easy, especially if it is burnt stubble. Sheep make tracks as well as people, and the route was not well marked at all. The grouse shooters were in evidence too, and I for one was very pleased that Jo's over-trousers were brilliant yellow.

The walk was the day before the annual 'Take Heart' Roundhay Park walk so I decided to miss it that year. Subsequently, I have been told that I was missed, so I have promised to participate in their next sponsored walk.

The transplant games in Portsmouth were enjoyable, but there were no medals for me that year. Transplant patients are surviving so much longer nowadays, particularly as the rejection drugs are so effective, and more veterans are well and active.

I had decided to enter tennis and table tennis, but no mini-marathon. I was practising tennis when I apparently tripped, Trying to get up off my bottom, I found that my left leg would not function. It was as if I had no muscle power at all, and my leg wobbled around like a rag doll. Helped off the court, I was attended to by a doctor on duty, and I feared the worst. However, after nearly an hour I was able to walk again, and even though I was told not to participate in any events, I played table tennis – being knocked out in the first round – walked the two miles, and ran the hundred metres. I walked a faster time this year and came fifth. Veterans start at forty-five years of age, and I can give them nearly twenty years, so in reality I cannot compete competitively.

Once again, the toddlers brought gasps of admiration and lumps to throats. Joan and Kevin joined us again for the Sunday, having decided to take a few days holidays in the area. Next year should be easier as the Games are in Sheffield. A very large, very colourfully dressed Jamaican lady came and sat next to us. Her eighteen-year-old son, who had had a heart transplant four years previously, was competing in some team events. His mother had come to the Games with most of her family. No sooner had this lady sat down than she was on her feet cheering on the competitors in a race. I asked her, "Is he. . ." indicating the leading runner, "from the hospital team?"

"No, my dear, I cheer everyone because all those taking part are winners."

How true.

While in Portsmouth, a visit to HMS *Victory* was arranged. As a child I had attended school in North Walsham, Norfolk, where Horatio Nelson had, for a short time, been a pupil at the boy's grammar school. On Trafalgar Day, October 21st, the boys, wearing black ties, went to the Parish Church and then had the rest of the day off as a holiday. The girls did not like this. The Queen Mother, when she was Queen, had on one occasion come to see Nelson's school, but we were informed that no High School girls were to be seen. A group of us, armed with school scarves, had sneaked out of our lesson and had received the royal wave. We were found out and duly seen to be punished by our sympathetic headmistress.

I enjoyed our visit to Victory, but would not have wanted to have been a member of its crew.

Alan and I decided to go into the New Forest since we were in the area, but as it was holiday time everyone else had the same idea. After crawling along for some time in the long line of traffic we decided to forget it and made for Lymington. This was teeming with people. However, it did bring back more childhood memories of reading Captain Marryat's *Children of the New Forest*.

On our return home I thought that maybe I should let the doctors at the hospital know of my collapsing leg. This meant extra trips to Leeds when various tests had been arranged. One test was a trans-oesophageal echocardiogram which involved having a tube down my throat. The letter received prior to the test stated that I should have a companion as I might feel drowsy. Joan, as usual, came with me.

I was given an injection in my wrist, and that's all I remember. I have no recollection of the test or dressing myself afterwards, or being told twice by the doctor and nurse that the test was satisfactory. Joan says that I almost ran to the railway station and she had to keep hold of my arm. On the train journey home I apparently sat opposite Joan, grinning inanely. When I mentioned my experience to Alison, she said that I would be a very good candidate for hypnosis.

An ultrasound test on my neck and a scan on my head also brought negative results. So ended the Portsmouth episode.

We had a welcome visit from our elder daughter, Cheryl, and her two sons, Matthew and Jonathan. Our two grandsons, who are both taller than me, communicate in grunts like so many teenage boys. It had been almost three years since we had last seen them, so we had a vast amount to catch up on.

Regular three monthly hospital visits continue and my fourth year MOT results were good. Each time I have been to Leeds recently one of the other transplantees has been an in-patient, so I have spent time with them. Hopefully they are now, once again, fit and well.

A few days before the end of term, Christmas 1994, I went into our local comprehensive school to talk to year ten pupils in science classes about heart transplants. One class sat silently for an hour, and when I asked the teacher if the talk had been all right, he said, "Did you see or hear anyone talking?"

"No," I hesitantly replied.

"Well, I've never known that lot stay quiet for so long."

I assumed from that comment that the lesson *was* satisfactory.

The other class asked several questions throughout the talk. One in particular surprised me. "How has your transplant affected you psychologically?" asked the boy.

"I don't think it has," I replied. "I know, though, that I am more tolerant and I certainly know what is important in life."

I was also asked if I carried a donor card for my new heart. I said no, because as far as I know my heart could not be used again, and my kidneys, liver, and lungs were probably damaged.

"Do you carry a card?" I asked the class. Do you, readers?

What of the future? I regard every day as a bonus and every day is wonderful whatever the weather.

I do find it difficult at times to believe that all this has happened to me. Out of the blue, I will suddenly think: Is it *all* a dream?

Alan and I tend not to plan too far ahead, but I do intend to live to see the year 2000 and beyond. Then, of course, there is still tap dancing!